D1488334

Becoming an Exceptional SLP Leader

14 Speech-Language Pathologists do More than Talk

With Foreword by Brian Goldstein, PhD, CCC-SLP

www.MaiLingChan.com

Mai Ling Chan, LLC

Phoenix, AZ

Table of Contents

Foreword

By Brian Goldstein, PhD

* * *

Everything looks like a failure in the middle . . . There are numerous roadblocks, obstacles, and surprises on the journey to change, and each one tempts us to give up. Give up prematurely, and the change effort is automatically a failure. Find a way around the obstacles, perhaps by making some tweaks in the plan, and keep going. Persistence and perseverance are essential to successful innovation and change.

~ Rosabeth Moss Kanter, the Ernest L. Arbuckle professor of business at Harvard Business School

At the intersection of individuality and communication lies one's voice. For my purposes here, one's *voice* has two meanings. Its first meaning relates to the way one communicates. That is, the mode might be via one's lungs, larynx, oral cavity, articulators, and other parts of the body, or it might be through augmentative or alternative means. The mode of communication is immaterial. What *is* material is the ability of all people to use any mode of communication in service to the message.

Communication, through the lens of speech-language pathology, is the focus of this outstanding volume edited by the incomparable Mai Ling Chan. She has assembled a talented, diverse, and accomplished group of speech-language pathologists (SLPs) to provide significance and illumination to the second meaning of *voice* –one's unique journey, style, and representation. Those voices are loud, clear, and distinctive, as evidenced by (some of) their own words:

Bilingual

Researcher

Minority

Storytelling

Diversity

First-generation

Identities

Accent

Challenge

Engage

Heritage

Reflection

Transformation

Sister, Brother, Mother, Father, Friend, Mentor, Colleague...

(Re)define

Lead

Opportunity

These authors provide a clarion call to all those who give their voice using any means of communication and those who communicate with exceptional individuals. Their voices and stories will resonate with all readers, myself included. I, too, have experienced that circuitous path, professionally and geographically–from theater major to linguistics major to practicing bilingual SLP to professor to researcher to academic leader–from South Carolina to Massachusetts to Pennsylvania to Missouri to New Jersey to California.

The authors' journeys serve to educate and inspire all of us, because their paths were neither preordained nor straightforward. They represent the vicissitudes inherent not only in communication and its development and use, but also in life. Their journeys, via their stories, coach us to be better and do better.

We are all what we are, in large degree, because of others who have helped, coached, taught, counseled, who set a standard by example, who've taken an interest in our interests, opened doors, opened our minds, helped us see, who gave encouragement when we needed it, who reprimanded or prodded when we needed it, and at critical moments, inspired.

~ David McCullough, author, narrator, popular historian, and lecturer

Finally, as did the chapter authors, I offer you the following:

Recommendations

1. You be you.
2. You do you.
3. Take an "I" position (see the work of psychiatrist Murray Bowen).
4. Extend grace to yourself and others.

Ways to Connect with Me

Twitter: @goldstein25

LinkedIn: https://tinyurl.com/46nvn36a

Brian Goldstein, PhD, CCC-SLP, is the chief academic officer and the executive dean of the College of Rehabilitative Sciences at the University of St. Augustine for Health Sciences. Based in San Marcos, Calif., his area of research focuses on speech sound development and disorders in Spanish-English bilingual children.

Acknowledgments

My family is my foundation. I thank my husband Cameron, and my children, Nick, Alex, and Raegan, for reminding me that joy abounds in the shared *experience*, not the achievement.

Thank you to my parents, Rosalba and Kan Chan, for listening to all of my dreams, opportunities, challenges, and disappointments. It's a roller coaster ride being my parent, but you're always right there beside me, with genuine excitement at the top and endless support at the bottom.

My deepest gratitude goes to each and every author for trusting the process and accepting my invitation to be vulnerable to inspire, guide, and support our colleagues and friends. Thank you for sharing with us. Your personal journey is precious, unique, and valued.

A special thanks to Pradeesh Thomas (CEO and cofounder, Verge Learning) and all of my partners and team members at Verge Learning and XceptionalED for matching my passion and commitment. I am proud to be a part of your team.

I could never have completed this book without you in my life: Matt Chan, Lori DiBlasi, Laura Stevenson, G. Patrick Poli, Thomas McDowell, Mary Huston, and my podcast hubby, Martyn Sibley.

Thank you for making it through all three books in this series with me! I am forever grateful to my amazing, international team of experts: Jennifer Baljko, developmental editor; Cori Wamsley, final editor; Christie Mayer, book cover; Jeren Calinisan, social media, and Angela Smith, content design. I can't imagine doing anything like this again without you.

Introduction

The final book in the *Becoming an Exceptional Leader* series spotlights a very unique niche of personal stories. In a broad sense, it is a collection of entrepreneurial and passion-focused leadership, spanning a wide range of interests, including but not limited to technology, research, clinical and staffing support, entertainment, and public service. But upon closer examination, each remarkable memoir has a unifying connection to the next: They weave together in the universally essential world of communication. Each author not only shares their intimate experiences as they moved through stages of progress, but they also invite you to explore your potential to serve on a larger scale and offer priceless insights to help expedite your development.

Each co-author has a history of professional service in the field of speech-language pathology. As reported by Arlene Pietranton, CEO of the American Speech-Language-Hearing Association (ASHA), in the ASHA CEO Update:[1]

May 2021, as of December 31, 2020, 188,143 members are reported to maintain the CCC-SLP certification (the Certificate of Clinical Competence, shortened to CCC is a nationally recognized professional credential representing a level of excellence in the field of speech-language pathology). It was a difficult task to include only 14 individuals to represent

---

[1] Pietranton, A. (2021, May). CEO Update May 2021. Retrieved September 20, 2021, from https://www.asha.org/about/governance/ceo-updates/ceo-update-may-2021/.

this impressive and highly accomplished community; however, I am confident that this is only one of many opportunities to spotlight the plethora of leaders in this field.

Similar to previous books in the *Becoming an Exceptional Leader* series, several authors were quite humble during our initial conversation and asked the question "What could I possibly share that would be helpful?" My reply was the same, "Anything you think would have helped you had you heard it earlier in your journey." Writing prompts helped the authors recall pivotal moments and dive deep into rediscovering their driving inspiration and daily motivation. I, too, tried to convey the mindset of my mentor Brené Brown, "to be the person who we long to be—we must again be vulnerable. We must take off the armor, put down the weapons, show up, and let ourselves be seen."[2]

As I read the first drafts of each chapter, I was overwhelmingly proud of how each author had embraced this style of writing—personal essay and memoir—and I was enamored with their eloquence and storytelling skills. Look beyond the intricate integration of depth and breadth of professional expertise with pure human experience and you'll see the underlying love of language that communicates their individual voices through the written word.

Although the majority of the chapters include the author's journey to pursue a career in speech-language pathology, the only commonality is that there isn't one. Many students identify their post-undergraduate path early on, but several

---

[2] Brown, Brené. *Daring Greatly: How the Courage to Be Vulnerable Transforms the Way We Live, Love, Parent, and Lead.* Avery, 2015.

authors demonstrate how a more winding road to the career can be just as fulfilling and impactful. It is our hope that our stories are shared across disciplines to inspire students to explore a career in communication disorders in order to help mitigate the severe shortage of professionals available to provide services. This is a global issue, and one that becomes increasingly more profound as the number of children and adults requiring services increases annually.

According to ASHA, "The speech-language pathologist (SLP) is defined as the professional who engages in professional practice in the areas of communication and swallowing across the lifespan. Communication and swallowing are broad terms encompassing many facets of function. Communication includes speech production and fluency, language, cognition, voice, resonance, and hearing. Swallowing includes all aspects of swallowing, including related feeding behaviors."[3]

The profession of speech-language pathology initially focused on elocution (clear and expressive speech) dating back to the 18th century in England. The field has since expanded to include highly focused domains of practice.

ASHA's Ad Hoc Committee on Service Delivery in the Schools developed the following guidelines and provided them as an official statement of the national organization, "A communication disorder is **an impairment in the ability to receive, send, process, and comprehend concepts or**

---

[3] American Speech-Language-Hearing Association. (2016) Scope of Practice in Speech-Language Pathology. Available from www.asha.org/policy

verbal, nonverbal and graphic symbol systems. A communication disorder may be evident in the processes of hearing, language, and/or speech. A communication disorder may range in severity from mild to profound."[4]

As you will read in the following chapters, the authors have achieved expertise in a wide variety of specialties including augmentative and alternative communication (AAC), stuttering, receptive and expressive language, and cognitive rehabilitation, to name a few. Their leadership extends beyond their clinical practice, building on foundational experiences, continued growth, dedication, and commitment. Creativity and courage are also at the heart of each story. This is evidenced by stories of international nonprofit creation, bilingualism, expansion to general education, public service, innovation, and entrepreneurism. But we are also easily united with the authors as they openly share personal battles with imposter syndrome, self-doubt, and fear of failure.

The term "exceptional" has been used in the title of this book series to reflect the gradual movement from the term "special needs" to "exceptional." Exceptional encompasses all deviation from the norm, for example, above or below average. The types of people who have been asked to share their stories with you glide towards "very much above average" in their internal compass, their driving force, their "why." Each Exceptional author was asked to include their personal inspiration in their chapter. THIS is the reason they

---

[4] Definitions of Communication Disorders and Variations. Ad Hoc Committee on Service Delivery in the Schools. https://www.asha.org/policy/rp1993-00208/

have worked so hard for so long. Whether their motivation and enthusiasm are linked to a person or an experience, the resulting impact is long-lasting and poignant

We invite you to share in our personal journeys and reflect on your own experiences. You may have already found your inspiration(s) and are ready to embark on the next step of your leadership path. We hope our recommendations are helpful to you, even if you've heard them all before. You never know when you will come across a pearl of wisdom that resonates with you on a deeper level, shifts your perspective, or reminds you of how exceptional you already are.

Most of all, we invite you to find joy in all that you do. Exceptional leadership mirrors your internal happiness. To quote co-author Amy Hill, M.S., CCC-SLP, "Do what you love, love what you do." What do you love?

Stop, Listen, and Collaborate

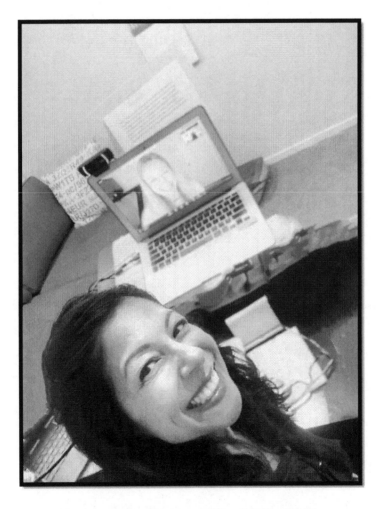

Mai Ling Chan, MS, CCC-SLP

* * *

It had been a busy morning, but I was able to get my nine-year-old son to his fourth grade classroom on time without remnants of breakfast on his face and my six-year-old to his first grade classroom with his special "All About My Family" poster intact.

Next up—my first clinical supervisor-attended therapy session for my master's program in speech-language pathology. As a returning student doing my grad work ten years post-baccalaureate, I had already experienced the anxiety and self-degradation that usually ensues when a student decides to re-enter the collegiate world, amplified by 100. Oh, and my program only accepted 35 stellar students from 500 national applicants. Yeah, no sweat! Ha!

Typical daily thoughts centered on, "How can I possibly compete with these kids?" and "How can I balance all the demands of school with being a homemade-lunch, fun-loving, always-available Super Mom?"

Curiously, this specific experience, a session with my supervisor looking on, wasn't adding to my normal level of stress. It was actually giving me the opportunity to display my studious nature and "people-skills"—or so I thought.

This was my first session with a client diagnosed with aphasia, which is a loss of ability to understand or express speech typically caused by brain damage. I carefully read through historical information, and after a thorough chart review, I created an activity that delved into a cueing hierarchy to identify target words. The task was straightforward, and I was pretty confident it would be effective for the 30-minute session. My client was an older gentleman who had suffered a stroke six months earlier. He had been attending the Arizona

State University Speech and Hearing Clinic for a few months already, working with students as they moved through their required clinical rounds. Upon arrival at the therapy room, he was very calm and friendly, and he and his wife both agreed to have my clinical supervisor attend the session via the two-way observation mirror in addition to videotaping the session for learning purposes.

Dr. Pamela Mathy, Ph.D., CCC-SLP, was not only my clinical supervisor for the semester but also the director of the Speech-Language Clinic at the time. I was quite honored to have the opportunity to have her guidance and expertise and was looking forward to receiving feedback on this session.

Adding to the smoothness of my morning, the session went exactly as planned, until it didn't. I opened the map of the United States and pointed to various states, providing a variety of carefully planned cues or "tips" to help my client identify each state. There were a few I thought were obvious like, "Everything's bigger in ___. " "It starts with T," and "T-e-x--." The client unfortunately struggled throughout the activity, and I felt helpless and enormously ineffective when he wasn't able to recall and verbalize the target word, for example, "Texas." But I pushed through nonetheless, hoping Dr. Mathy would look past this and instead recognize my thoroughness in integrating the cueing hierarchy throughout the session, eventually resulting in a few successful state identifications.

When the session ended, I thanked my client and wife, and met Dr. Mathy in a nearby room where she had already set up the DVD for review. She had it cued to about 15 minutes from the start and told me to watch for about 10 minutes when she would return and we could discuss it together.

I was quite excited and pressed play.

As I watched myself sitting next to the older gentleman, I immediately noticed a few unforgettable details: My posture was stiff and unyielding, with an almost aggressive nature as I passionately pointed to the map on the table in front of us and used overt hand gestures. My facial features were determined and serious while my words were relentless and unabating. In contrast, the gentleman was hunched over with his head lowered somewhat. He shook his head "no" periodically as he struggled to retrieve and say the target word. He took deep breaths and sighed once in a while. At one point, he looked at me and smiled, almost as if to say, "I'm sorry. I really want to do this for you, but I just can't." I was stunned.

Dr. Mathy returned and found me with tears streaming down my face. I was so ashamed, so embarrassed by how I had choreographed the entire session to be ABOUT ME, and not once focused on the fellow human I was with. I can't remember exactly what Dr. Mathy said because my mind was swimming with shame but I remember this phrase—"like a bull in a china closet," referring to my aggressive use of word retrieval supports in the delicate clinical space. It was at that moment that I promised myself to always put my own ego and initiatives aside and focus on the person I was supporting.

This one experience forever changed how I entered into clinical interactions. It also helped to transform my personal and professional growth. The first crucial step I saw I needed to take was learning how to stop talking so much, and listen more. This meant listening to what the other person was saying as well as not saying, and watching their body language. I began biting on my back teeth during sessions and increasing "wait time" (a period of time without cueing, hints, or feedback to allow a client to process and formulate responses) to what felt like an eternity to me. I remember breaking out in full sweats during these early trials, fighting with myself to stay silent and honor the space in between all the words.

Eventually, what started out as tortuous and foreign, slowly began to become more comfortable and natural. I noticed, too, how I was able to incorporate this technique into my parenting style as well as personal and professional relationships. Of course, my little brother would argue that I still "don't listen," but I jokingly argue that he's typically wrong and so his opinion doesn't count (even though I've adored him since the moment he came into my life when I was 12 years old).

In all seriousness, I have found such joy in active listening that this has truly become the inspiration for much of my work since achieving my degree and becoming a speech-language pathologist over 15 years ago. As a clinician, I have served clients across different ages and settings, including preschool, K–12 school and home settings, acute and long-term rehabilitation, home health, and memory care. Throughout the years, I have met many amazing people and have learned so much from their personal stories shared during our time together. I am definitely the type of person who takes her clients home with her—sharing successes and fun anecdotes with my family during dinner (names and locations protected, of course). My kids, adults now, have even surprised me once in a while by asking, "How are those twins you used to work with?" or "Remember the patient who had the stroke and you saved his kitten?" (a story for another day).

I have also loved listening to the stories of my colleagues and other people who are committed to supporting people with disabilities. This is where my work has been focused during the past few years.

My entrepreneurial career in the disability community began in 2012 after reading in-depth blog posts reviewing software apps being implemented for speech therapy. I was amazed by how thorough the reviews were and loved the specific clinical-use cases and stories of personal experiences. This sparked my idea to ask all speech-language pathologists (SLPs) which apps they recommended, and together, we created a Yelp-like review site for speech therapy apps. Through this experience, I learned the beauty and power of collaboration, which has also become a foundational cornerstone of my work.

Since then, my focus has been on spotlighting people all over the world who have dedicated their lives to making a difference for people with disabilities. Branching out from speech therapy apps, I connected with remarkable SLPs who dedicated countless hours to sharing their clinical expertise through priceless blog posts and in-person presentations and invited them to create and sell online courses. I used words like "branding," "audience," and "product"— terms not readily used in our service industry, and many clinicians were interested and excited to create a course, but they weren't ready to "market and sell" their courses online.

Truthfully, back in 2018, even as the online course option drew attention, SLPs weren't really enthralled about learning online. Although the concept of a marketplace of courses dedicated to speech-language pathology was novel and valuable, building our online professional development company was slow and seriously restricted because my co-founders and I all worked full-time jobs and simply couldn't dedicate the hours and brainpower required to grow and *scale* from a small side gig to a real startup. And although I was investing my own capital to keep the minimal financial overhead maintained, I didn't believe enough in its actual potential to leave my j-o-b and go "all-in."

But, this didn't mean I wasn't still listening.

In 2018, I learned about the world of audio content while listening to the awe-inspiring guests on Oprah Winfrey's *Super Soul Sunday* and NPR journalist Guy Raz's *How I Built This* shows. I loved the ability to hear them and their guests actually speaking and the intimate feeling of sitting right there at the table with them as they talked. This was a whole new level up from the blog experience, and I wanted to be the person asking the questions and *listening* to my guest's inspiring answers!

I was so excited by the idea of creating a show that would spotlight inspiring people in the disability community that I literally Google-searched and met with Evo Terra, one of the authors of the internationally recognized yellow and black covered book "Podcasting for Dummies," who also happened to live 30 minutes away from me in Phoenix, Arizona. I was quickly connected with a local audio engineer and started a podcast spotlighting one person a week via a 45-minute interview-style show. My sensational audio engineer is still with me more than three years and 100+ episodes later, and I am now joined by my co-host, Martyn Sibley, a highly recognized United Kingdom-based disability leader. Together we have reached over 52 countries, sharing the stories of people who are making a difference in the world for people with disabilities. (You can read his story in the first book of this series, *Becoming an Exceptional Leader.*)

Around the same time, Lucas Steuber, MS, CCC-SLP (another amazing SLP Leader who shared his story in the second book in this series, *Becoming an Exceptional AAC Leader*) reached out to me to see if there was a way to collaborate and support the fascinating speech therapy-focused podcast shows he had recently created with Matt Hott Matthew Hott MS, CCC-SLP (read his chapter on page 73); Rachel Madel, MS, CCC-SLP (read her chapter on page 114); and Chris Bugaj, MS, CCC-SLP. Along with our start-up team, we created a small network of shows, providing marketing and branding support and organizing occasional sponsorship income. Although we have since disbanded, I am honored to have been a part of the Speech Science and Talking With Tech podcast teams, and am so proud of all of the people who worked together to make the episodes come to life and reach enormous global audiences.

Somewhere during my first 50 solo podcast interviews, I realized that my audience was limited to people who listened to podcasts. While the number of podcast listeners has been steadily increasing over the years, in 2018 only 26% of people in the U.S. were listening.[5] To extend the reach of my podcast guests, I decided to unite their stories within the classic

[5] Edison Research and Triton Digital. "The Infinite Dial 2021." http://www.edisonresearch.com/wp-content/uploads/2021/03/The-Infinite-Dial-2021.pdf

medium of the written word, which marked the beginning of the three-book anthology series, *Becoming an Exceptional Leader, Becoming an Exceptional AAC Leader*, and this final edition, *Becoming an Exceptional SLP Leader.* Each book has been a beautiful collaboration of extraordinary people who have entrusted me and my editorial team to share their stories with the world, and the feedback has been astoundingly rewarding. When people ask me if it's worth writing a book, I tell them that the monetary rewards are minimal, but the connection with your readers is priceless.

The rewarding connection with our audience, readers, and people in our everyday lives has shown in other ways, too. Along those lines, I can also share good news about the professional development platform my co-founders and I created at XceptionalED, the company we started in 2018.

Although it was slow growing, the presenters we supported in speech-language pathology and assistive technology also advanced in their own expertise, course-creation skills, and online presence, so our course sales and brand recognition increased—and people were noticing. In August, 2020, we connected with a new special education-focused digital content and teletherapy company looking to grow by partnering with an established company. By this time, we had already had a good amount of experience with pitching and "dating" possible investment partners, and approached this opportunity with tempered enthusiasm. After a long process of interviews with all major stakeholders in both companies, our XceptionalEd start-up team unanimously agreed to move forward, and we announced our acquisition by Verge Learning in January 2021.

It was a bumpy transition, merging two established companies and personnel, but we learned each other's best practices, established new processes, and successfully became one team serving children and special education teams all over the world.

After about six months, I decided to take the leap of faith and work full time for our newly merged company. Although I was initially torn over missing the opportunity to continue creation and research with the assistive technology team I had been working with for the past year, I was very excited to commit to my start-up team and be able to focus on our company every day, all day. I can honestly say that this has been an absolute joy for me. I am now able to integrate all of my clinical experience, technical knowledge, business acumen, entrepreneurial spirit, passion, and positive attitude into everything I do to serve my global community of partners, teammates, course and content creators, colleagues, parents, and ultimately, students who benefit from special education support.

The most important piece of what I have shared is the fact that I have never been alone.

Beginning with Dr. Mathy's honest and invaluable feedback, I have continued to grow and learn from all of the professionals I have clinically worked with, phenomenal course presenters, podcast guests, glowing reviews and occasional criticism received from the previous books, book and podcast teammates, and all of my precious start-up team members who have worked alongside me through several of my BHAGs (big, hairy, audacious goals). There is no way I could have widened my ripple in the world without each and every person who has come into my life and joined me on my journey. And, each stop along the way presents a new opportunity to stop, *listen*, and collaborate.

Recommendations

1. **Watch for the learning moments in your life.** They can come when you least expect them.
2. **Be open to opportunities to work together with others.** They can be in an area of interest, profession, or even personal circles.
3. **Actively listen in all situations**. For some people, this is very natural, and for others, we have to really work on being fully present and less egocentric.
4. **Don't allow negative feedback to overwhelm you.** Accept constructive criticism and release yourself from trying to please everyone all the time.

My Wish for You

In previous chapters of the *Becoming an Exceptional Leader* book series, I shared my personal struggles with word-finding, perfectionism, and imposter syndrome when compared with fellow co-authors. In this chapter, I share clinical service immaturity, lessons learned, and progress through collaboration. Through my podcast interviews and coordinating this book series, I have learned that although EVERYONE experiences and handles challenges in their own unique ways (even those who see them as "opportunities" and have the "challenge accepted!" attitude), ultimately, these life experiences help to shape and stretch you beyond your comfort zone, further open your heart and mind, and increase your optimum reach and effect on the world. I hope that if you experience a few of these struggles, they will be less painful and that you have good resources (like this book), wonderful mentors, and effective strategies to move through or mitigate them with greater ease and early success.

My Community

Listen to my episode on the Xceptional Leaders podcast:

https://bit.ly/mai_ling_chan

Mouse over the QR code with your phone's photo app open to go directly to the podcast.

Ways to Connect with Me

www.mailingchan.com

Twitter: https://twitter.com/mailingchan

LinkedIn: https://www.linkedin.com/in/mailingchan

Facebook: https://www.facebook.com/MaiLingChanSLP

Clubhouse: @mailingchanSLP

Mai Ling Chan is a speech-language pathologist, author, publisher, business consultant, and international speaker. In addition to her position as co-founder and chief of partnerships with Verge Learning, she also co-hosts the Xceptional Leaders Podcast, and is an original co-founder of XceptionalED.

At the Heart of Making a Difference

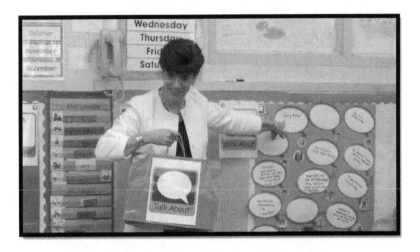

Phyl Macomber, MS ATP

Photographer: Beltrami Studios

* * *

We all have many commemorative moments in our lives.

Commemorative moments are occasions that mark a life transition, milestones and important events, such as your graduation day or the day you start a new job and embark on a new career. These are certainly memorable times in life.

In my own professional life, one of my commemorative moments was the day I began my clinical fellowship at Johns Hopkins Hospital's Kennedy Krieger Institute.

Back then, in 1988, when it was named Kennedy Institute for Handicapped Children, I gazed up at the famous Johns Hopkins dome for the first time and was awestruck by the idea of working under the very roof where new syndromes and medical treatments were being discovered on a regular basis. From training pediatric residents to serving families who traveled internationally for answers to their children's challenges, beginning my career in zip code 21287 on North Broadway in Baltimore, Md., was most definitely a commemorative moment in my life.

There are other types of moments, however, that I would like to chat with you about: They are called "defining" moments. A defining moment is a time when life presents you with the opportunity to make a *pivotal decision*. It is when you experience something that **fundamentally changes you**. These types of moments enable you to hone in on your *greatest talents* so you can make your *greatest contributions*. And, trust me, you will not have any trouble identifying a defining moment when it happens to you because it will empower you to take action and create a positive turning point in your life, from which you will draw endless motivation and inspiration.

Defining moments help you uncover your passion and figure out what matters to you. They help put you on a purposeful path so you can make a difference to help others.

I am 60 years old, and have served in the field of education since 1988. Many defining moments have put me on courses I never could have imagined, both personally and professionally. These defining moments have helped me figure out *my* true passion, which is setting up inclusive systems of learning so every child can learn, reach their true potential, and make meaningful contributions when learning new information and sharing what they know in their classroom community.

I firmly believe that a child does not "earn" their way into the general education classroom. *It is that child's fundamental right to be there*. It is a child's right to be a contributing member of their classroom community. It is a child's right to be a contributing member of their school community. It is also a child's right for their contributions to have purpose and personal significance.

I learned this firsthand as a child from my Aunt Nellie and Uncle Sammy, parents of my cousin Pam, who has an intellectual disability. By example, the two of them defined inclusion for me as a child in the early 1960s. Aunt Nellie taught me that inclusion centered on contributions; being given the *opportunity* to make a contribution and one that was *meaningful*.

For example, every Columbus Day weekend, my paternal grandfather Pop-Pop, made wine, just like he did back in Italy before he took the boat to Ellis Island. All of us cousins stomped on the grapes and used the wine press. Pam was right there with us, with everyone turning varying shades of purple! Then, during cousins' birthday parties, we all loved jumping on the bed listening to the Monkees—Pam often leading the charge. It was not "us" and "her" . . . Pam was a part of "we."

As the author of T.H.E. P.A.C.T., a research-based teaching framework, and the CEO of Make A Difference Inc., I have taken my knowledge in the field of speech-language pathology, along with my co-teaching experiences with teachers, and provided a solution to a series of problems with which I see educators continually struggle.

Teaching staff have days filled with multiple things to do and simply not enough time to do them. In addition, educators are faced with attempting to cover an incredible amount of information in an unrealistic and often impossible amount of time. Although we have individualized education plans in place "on paper" for our students receiving specialized instruction, teams continue to struggle with delivering purposeful instruction and meaningful inclusion from preschool to high school.

As opposed to feeling overwhelmed, it was important to me that educators could feel good about their daily contributions and *reach students of all abilities*. I knew that the answer was to systemize instruction in a delivery model that could be used by *all* teaching staff: classroom teachers, special educators, therapists, and consultants, therefore bridging the gap between special education and general education. This teaching framework helps staff focus, organize, and streamline their time so they can maximize their impact and use their time wisely. In addition, it does not have an expiration date, meaning it can be used from preschool through graduation.

In 2009, if you were to ask me if I would ever embark on such a journey as I am on now to make an impact in education, I would have smiled at you and thought you were bonkers! I did, however, have a defining moment occur in Orlando, Fla. that put me on this very path in the winter of 2009.

I was presenting educational sessions with a colleague at the Assistive Technology Industry Association (ATIA) national conference in January of that year. During the conference, Meg Turek, the managing editor of the *Closing The Gap Solutions* publication, approached me about writing an article for their educational publication.

I looked at Meg and said, "You want *me* to write an article? What would I possibly write about, Meg?"

She looked at me affectionately and replied, "Phyl, I want you to write about something you are passionate about and something that matters to you. I want you to share your voice."

And so it began.

On the plane ride back to New England, I examined what truly mattered to me in education. I was very passionate about simplifying learning, which, in turn, would simplify teaching. This defining moment birthed the publication of a 4-step, color-coded teaching framework that I created, called T.H.E. P.A.C.T., which is an acronym that stands for *Technology Helps Easy and Practical Accessible Curriculum Teaching*. It is a "common sense" approach for teaching students from gifted to special needs–and every student in between. T.H.E. P.A.C.T. provides a practical blueprint for Universal Design for Learning (UDL) instruction in any setting.

My article focused on adapting curriculum and making curriculum content accessible for all students with varying disabilities in the classroom setting. My speech-language background served as my compass for creating this framework. Over the years, one of my core objectives was to encourage educators to partner with the language specialists in their buildings; such a partnership, I believed, was crucial to the academic success of all students because "curriculum *is* language."

After the article appeared in 2009, I published my first book, recorded and produced educational resources, launched national training tours for seminars on my framework, and presented six educational sessions on T.H.E. P.A.C.T. at various national conferences.

My project started with a simple vision and heartfelt hope that it would make an impact. Over time, I saw those efforts grow and become effective in different parts of the world— across North America in the United States and Canada, in various countries in Africa, and in parts of Australia, Italy, England, and Saudi Arabia.

At the heart of it all for me is to honor what my dear parents taught me in life: the importance of making a difference with purpose-driven service.

Believe me when I say to you, though, that the scale of this project was *way out of my comfort zone.*

The 2013–2014 school year was an academic year of tremendous growth for T.H.E. P.A.C.T. I consulted with and trained special educators, classroom teachers, therapists, and specialists on how best to instruct their students receiving special education services in the general education classroom. Lines of communication opened up between school staff, administrators, and of equal significance, the parents. I was thrilled when classroom teachers found the framework's strategies highly effective for not only their students receiving specialized instruction, but also successful *with their entire class.*

This was another defining moment for me, and it was one of immense gratitude related to fostering inclusive practices in education. Yet, it was also a moment of feeling extremely overwhelmed regarding the road ahead of me. I felt I was being pulled in so many different directions. Principals were contacting me to conduct school-wide initiatives. I served on numerous strategic planning committees with directors of curriculum. I spoke with school boards, presented at numerous national conferences a year, and began a research study in nineteen locations across the United States and Canada. I also became an app developer on a moment's notice.

My days were filled with meetings with teacher after teacher—some wanting to learn and others just showing up because they were told they "had to do it" by their administrator. Some days, I felt as if I was in my favorite movie, *The Wizard of Oz*, running from the flying monkeys and not seeing a clear path to the Emerald City. I had many restless nights and countless mornings when I was at my desk at 4:00 a.m. I had so many spinning plates, and I was just waiting for them to all come crashing down.

And they did. It was the fall of 2013, Wednesday, October 30, to be precise. I remember it like it was yesterday. It was my husband Rob's birthday, and he came home to find me sitting in my grandfather's barber chair in our living room in Vermont on a chilly evening. The fireplace was blazing, and I was drinking a cup of tea, my favorite, *Taylors of Harrogate Yorkshire Gold* with lemon. I was sobbing.

Rob immediately came over to comfort me and frantically asked me what had happened. My father's health had recently started to decline, so Rob thought my emotional state was related to news about my dad.

I looked up at my husband with tears streaming down my cheeks and said, "I have lost my 'WHY' . . . and the joy in my work, Partner." I burst into tears again. Uncontrollably. "Rob, I am not sure that I can get it back. That is what I am most worried about."

Rob looked at me lovingly and kissed me on the forehead. He walked into my study and came back into the living room holding a copy of my first published article on T.H.E. P.A.C.T. from 2009, the one Meg Turek had asked me to write. He said, "Read this, Little Girl. You haven't lost your WHY. You just need to be reminded of it."

I read through the article, page after page, about "why" I created T.H.E. P.A.C.T. and why it was important to help children achieve their true potential. This was THE defining moment in my life, the one that clarified the work I was meant to do in the world and the contributions that were mine to offer.

The two-hour conversation with Rob on his birthday that year fundamentally changed me. I was reminded of what I knew about myself all along: I am an advocate for children with disabilities. I will remain tireless in my efforts to empower educators with meaningful inclusionary practices. I also know that I am successful doing a handful of things and doing them well. In fact, this is a foundational principle of T.H.E. P.A.C.T. framework that I authored. It was a pivotal point for me, which resulted in me not saying "yes" to everything moving forward because I felt that I needed to serve to the point of exhaustion.

I started to make more responsible decisions . . . those that gave me joy and made me 100% passionate about pursuing. I trusted my gut when approached with an idea or a request for service. I got rid of things that drained my energy. I also made time for myself—to grow, to learn, and to develop professional skills in other areas I never would have thought of before, such as formal training in speaking to the media or specific business principles that could help catapult my project.

Now, as a result of that awareness and setting healthy boundaries, I only mentor and coach people who want to learn and want to better serve in education and the business world. I focus on "My Vital Three," the short list of top priorities, for a specific time period and get them across the finish line. I am working "smarter, not harder" by archiving recorded seminars so people can learn on their own time and on their own schedule. I also redefined the focus of my philanthropic contributions, which gives me a great deal of gratification.

I dabble in other aspects of my project that give me joy: writing my new book series, being a regular guest on radio programs and talk shows to have purposeful conversations about education, and donating time to international organizations, such as serving on the Board of Directors for the *Leave No Girl Behind School of Leadership*, based in South Africa. **These are things that really matter to me.**

My parents always taught me that no contribution was too little and that every effort to help someone counted in life. October 30, 2013 was a defining moment in my life when I was at my low . . . when I called *everything* into question. It was a game-changer for me to turn it around and be successful at making a better difference in my purpose-driven service.

I now write to you with tears in my eyes, because one year later, on October 30, 2014, on my husband's birthday, I buried my greatest teacher in life—my Daddy. As I reflect on the serendipity of this, I realize there is much truth to the saying, "You do not know how strong you are until you have to be strong."

I have had, and continue to have, many defining moments and real-life struggles throughout the growth of my educational project. These defining moments have served as sharpening stones for me, both as a professional and as a human being.

As I look to the future, I embrace each challenge with eagerness and enthusiasm. I never lose sight of why I do what I do. My moral compass always points to my belief that every child can learn and that I can be a change agent in education.

Recommendations

As a result of all of my experiences on my Yellow Brick Road of Life, I share these personal recommendations with you to serve as "Your Vital Three" when making a difference:

1. **Indict the status quo.** You can make a better difference in the lives of the people you serve by not being afraid of indicting the status quo. You need to have the courage to challenge the existing state of affairs when the current model, or parts of the current model, are not working. You do this by calling into question that which is broken, flawed to begin with, or simply flat-out wrong.

2. **Examine your belief system and stay true to your passion.** Use *your* belief system as a moral compass each day that you serve. It is all about the contribution, paying it forward, making an impact, and helping

others. Never lose the fire in your belly for purpose-driven service.

3. **Know your why.** As a part of this process, answer the question, "What is *your* WHY?" Because if you know your "WHY"—truly know it and believe in it—you will get others to believe in it, too.

My Wish for You

My heartfelt wish for you is to believe that as long as you want to make a difference, you will find your own unique way to do so. My hope for you is that you will adopt the practice of self-reflection to grow and change as a person and as a professional.

We have the power to change anything. I wish to empower you to take steps to shape and shift belief systems through your own creative ideas of how you can help others.

Remember . . .

"No matter who you are,

No matter what you do . . .

YOU have the power to change *anything*."

- Phyl Macomber

My Community

Listen to my interview on the Xceptional Leaders Podcast with Mai Ling Chan:

https://bit.ly/phyl_macomber

Mouse over the QR code with your phone's photo app open to go directly to the podcast.

Ways to Connect with Me

Website:
AboutTHEPACT.com

Email:
Phyl@AboutTHEPACT.com

Facebook:
https://www.facebook.com/phylmacomber/ and
https://www.facebook.com/phyl.thepact

Twitter: https://twitter.com/AllAboutTHEPACT

LinkedIn: https://www.linkedin.com/in/phylthepact/

Phyl Macomber is the CEO of Make a Difference Inc. She is an award-winning speaker, bestselling author, and education specialist who has trained thousands of educators around the globe, advocating for children of all abilities to reach their potential in an inclusive environment. Phyl's Amazon #1 bestseller *Every Child Can Learn: Your Roadmap to Inclusive Education* is being referred to as "common sense education" by educators around the world.

A Career Rediscovered!

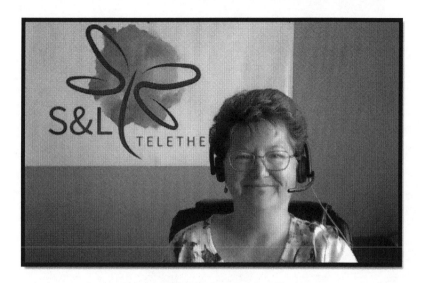

Tracy Sippl, MS, CCC-SLP

* * *

Love of teaching runs in my family. My grandmother, aunt, and sister each taught for over 20 years. I would play "school" with my friends, using the workbooks my grandmother gave me when they went out of print and were no longer used at the school where she taught.

In the mid-1980s when my grandmother suffered a series of strokes stealing her ability to express her thoughts, ideas, and needs, I shifted my focus to communication disorders. I was an undergraduate student at the University of Wisconsin-Madison at the time and worked to develop a very basic communication board my grandmother could use to help her express her needs.

While completing my clinical practicum, I worked with children in a school-based setting, and that's where I fell in love with speech-language pathology.

I graduated with my bachelor's degree in 1987 and a master's degree in 1989, both from UW-Madison. After my second child was born, I became interested in implementing technology during service delivery using an iPod and then eventually transitioned to an iPad. My son's growing interest in technology had me wondering whether technology could be used to strengthen educational skills. The internet was finally becoming available where I lived, even though it was dial up and connecting took forever! I began researching educational websites, games, and applications that piqued my son's interest, and realized that some could be used to practice skills and strategies taught in speech-language therapy.

In the early 2000s, educational computer games came to market, and I explored ways to use them to supplement my in-person therapy. As the internet landed in schools, I began to use educational websites to supplement my therapy materials and generalize skills. Students were engaged and excited by the variety of materials I used to teach and practice strategies as well as practicing speech skills. I eventually also incorporated music, movement, videos, and games for positive reinforcement as well as a multi-modality approach to therapy.

When I first began considering telepractice in 2011, it was not widely accepted by many companies or school districts. As a matter of fact, one of the myths about telepractice was that the quality of services provided in this manner was *less* than that of in-person services. Telepractice was thought of as "Plan B" and was only to be implemented when necessary.

What drew me to telepractice were the advantages it afforded such as working from home, making my own schedule, and using my creativity when pulling together hard-copy and online materials for my students. I liked the challenge of changing people's minds. The more I researched how therapy services could be delivered via telepractice, I knew I could provide the quality of services necessary and make it even more engaging than in-person services. After all, what student wouldn't like to work on tasks using a video-conferencing platform while interacting with online materials? My own son found video games so engaging. Why couldn't therapy be the same?

Honestly, though, I considered becoming a telepractitioner for a more personal reason.

I was diagnosed with fibromyalgia and chronic fatigue syndrome in 2000. While I had fought my hardest to work in-person, my body was failing me. I was exhausted all the time, and my body was in constant pain, so much so that I could hardly focus on my job.

I quit working in schools and opened my own private practice, running it out of my home from 2000 to 2004. During that time, I worked with a number of naturopathic physicians to get my symptoms under control. By 2005, I felt ready to go back into the schools.

I was able to work part-time for a number of years, but I slowly began experiencing severe symptoms once again in 2011 due to the stress at work, keeping up a busy schedule, and raising my children. I realized that I was not able to give

100% to my students and family and have a life, simultaneously. Something had to change.

Around the same time, a travel-therapy company contacted me. The company was interested in piloting a telepractice program, and they asked if I would like to work with them in developing the program and providing services to a group of students. I accepted, and the next thing I knew, I was on a plane to a telepractice training program in Maine! After that training, my mind was made up! I was going to dive into telepractice head-first.

I remember working with my first telepractice student. The platform was clunky, and the internet connection waxed and waned at times. I found myself having to repeat what I just said or asking the client to do the same, but making telepractice fun and exciting was easy because I was thrilled to have the opportunity to use it! My clients were excited to actually be able to use a computer to "go to speech therapy." I remember, on one occasion, my client laughing so hard he was gasping for air. The screen had frozen and my face was contorted while I had been talking—that was the frozen image on his screen! His laughter made me laugh, as I could only imagine what my frozen face looked like on his computer! When I use the video-conferencing platforms now and compare them to when I first began providing telepractice services, the technology *now* leaves the past in the dust! Frozen screens (and faces) are basically a thing of the past (thank goodness).

In time, I reached out to a few established telepractice companies and expanded my telepractice services. I ended up working with three different therapy companies at the same time (I wouldn't recommend this to anyone). I found myself working approximately 50-60 hours a week, which was crazy! Besides having to learn the different video-conferencing platforms each company used, I also had to learn how to enter data into each school district's documentation system.

I encountered other challenges when I began providing telepractice services.

For example, telepractice companies often did not set up expectations with school districts and/or parents of virtual-education students. During one contract, I was required to provide telepractice services to Pre-K students in the back of their classroom while the other students played and participated in "Circle Time." In another instance, while working with students attending a virtual academy, students were serviced from home with siblings and parents talking and yelling to each other in the background not realizing that I could hear them. Or, students competed for Wi-Fi bandwidth with siblings or parents watching Netflix, for example. And, when I worked with a virtual academy, the Individualized Education Plan (IEP) team would frequently forget to invite me to the meetings.

It was also difficult to help parents and school district administration understand that telepractice is only a different type of service delivery model, not a different type of service. On top of that, there was also a lack of respect from other professionals and SLPs (speech language pathologists) who had little to no knowledge of what "telepractice" was.

Frequently, too, parents and/or teachers were only made aware that the child was receiving *virtual* SLP services while attending an IEP meeting; introductory emails were never sent out by the school district as promised (now, as a result, I email parents and teachers directly *myself*).

Of course, there were technology issues as well. Some schools' Wi-Fi was taxed during specific times of the day, which greatly impacted telepractice service delivery. Wi-Fi is *much better* now, but back then, the screen would consistently freeze or the connection would often drop when the school's computer lab was in use.

And, finally, changing perceptions about telepractice took time and attention. Some SLPs believed that telepractice was just sitting down in front of a computer and "doing" therapy. Those who did were in for a rude awakening, if that was their expectation, a point driven home during the Covid-19 pandemic when telepractice became the norm.

In time, I reduced my workload and worked with two telepractice companies at a time. They would only offer part-time work, and I wanted something that would give me a specific number of hours, more than just one company was willing to give.

In 2017, Mai Ling Chan reached out to me about doing a live interview to discuss telepractice. I was so nervous! The more we chatted during the interview, the more confident I became as I remembered the variety of experiences I had in providing telepractice. I was excited to share information with others about the exciting prospect of providing therapy using this other service delivery model.

Because I ended up having to "figure out" telepractice on my own, I created continuing education courses about telepractice, something Mai Ling encouraged me to do. I wanted to help people develop a thorough understanding of what "telepractice" was. Since telepractice was just beginning to gain national attention in our field of work, information was not always readily available about being HIPAA (Health Insurance Portability and Accountability Act of 1996) compliant and maintaining confidentiality. I wanted to help people learn how to set up their home offices, debunk myths about telepractice, and self-advocate during a telepractice interview. I love everything telepractice and was thrilled to be able to share the information!

In 2018, I was elected to American Speech-Language-Hearing Association's (ASHA) Special Interest Group (or SIG) 18: Telepractice Coordinating Committee and was honored to represent individuals providing telepractice services because the committee only had one other person who could actually speak to providing telepractice services firsthand.

While serving on the SIG18: Telepractice Coordinating Committee, we would hear on social media about what people were doing while providing remote therapy, such as servicing clients while traveling the country in an RV, wearing pajamas during telepractice, having a backdrop of a bed covered with piles of miscellaneous items and/or laundry, nursing a baby while providing services...and this was before Covid-19 hit! I made it my mission to address ethical considerations when providing telepractice services and that continues even today.

Looking back, I realize that I could not find a mentor to answer my questions about how to begin. Rarely did the telepractice company have someone to address telepractice questions. I usually ended up speaking with the recruiter who had little knowledge about the actual service delivery. How would I know if telepractice was right for me? What equipment was required? What questions should I ask a telepractice company?

Around 2016, I was receiving and responding to a multitude of Facebook requests about telepractice, and it dawned on me that other SLPs were experiencing the same lack of mentorship. I was also more frequently being invited to speak to state, national, and international associations about telepractice as this was still fairly new to the professional population.

That's when I decided to start my own consulting company, and S&L Teletherapy Consulting, LLC was born!

When Covid-19 hit and schools shut down, there was an outcry for information about telepractice. Many were thrust into the telepractice world without any preparation. School districts reached out to me, asking about training their "in-person" SLPs to do telepractice. SLPs contacted me asking about what they needed to know to provide telepractice services.

Today, you'll see posts on Facebook from those who fell in love with telepractice and those who did not (they could not wait to go back to in-person services). My heart went out to all of those SLPs who were required to provide a hybrid approach. I cannot imagine what they went through trying to serve their large caseloads with some students being seen in-person and preparing those materials while others were serviced via telepractice.

As many people adjust to providing telepractice services during the ebb and flow of the pandemic, I can say now with the wisdom of hindsight that my physical challenges over the years led me down a path that I had never thought about before: using technology to provide speech-language pathology services.

When I thought that I would have to end my SLP career to manage my health issues, telepractice helped me realize that I could continue to work with students using a different type of service delivery model. Telepractice allowed me to use a *different* method of service delivery, one that would allow me to set my own schedule, work from home, have a life outside of work, and be my own boss.

During my journey, I have learned that I am strong and driven, and that I can also demonstrate self-care. I also learned that being an SLP was not an all-or-nothing career (work in-person or you don't work at all). By connecting with others, working with students, and offering advice and information to other SLPs about telepractice, I knew I wasn't alone. I could connect with other SLPs with the click of a button. That realization was both liberating and empowering!

Recommendations

1. **Stay connected.** Telepractice can be isolating, so be sure to make connections and keep them current. Reach out to others even if just to say, "Hello!"
2. **Have confidence in your clinical abilities.** Believe in yourself and your skills. If you know you lack experience in a specific area (for instance, telepractice), seek out the training necessary to put your best foot forward when servicing clients.
3. **Be gentle with yourself.** Telepractice, as any new skill, has a learning curve. Be sure to take time to research, learn, and practice the skills necessary for quality service delivery.

4. **Ease in to telepractice.** If you aren't sure you want to switch from in-person services to strictly telepractice, try providing telepractice services part-time. When I first began, I worked in-person 60% of the time and during my days off, I provided telepractice until I knew I wanted to provide telepractice services full time.

5. **Try not to lose sight of what telepractice is and is <u>not</u>**. It is not about the "bells and whistles" or green screens. Telepractice, as therapy in general, should be 100% client-focused, and the online games and websites should <u>supplement</u> your services, <u>not be the focus</u>.

My Wish for You

As I have worked through my health and career challenges, I have come to realize a number of things.

First, don't give up. If people tell you, "You can't," know that you *can*. Many times, challenges will push you in unanticipated directions.

Second, be mindful of your personal needs. Self-care goes a long way to help avoid career burnout. Take care of yourself and your needs. This will allow you to continue to serve others.

Lastly, keep believing. I have a screensaver on my phone that reminds me daily who is in control of everything. I love starting my day out with this: *Pray. Then let it go. Don't try to force it or manipulate the outcome. Just trust God to open the right doors at the right time.*

(https://www.facebook.com/SpeakLifeQuotes/).

My Community

Watch my interview with Mai Ling Chan on YouTube:

https://bit.ly/tracy_sippl1

Mouse over the QR code with your phone's photo app open to go directly to the interview.

Ways to Connect with Me

www.s-lteletherapyconsulting.com

Facebook:
https://www.facebook.com/teletherapyconsulting/

Instagram: @slteletherapyconsulting

Besides being a wife and mother of two adult children, Tracy Sippl, MS, CCC-SLP, is a licensed, American Telemedicine Association Program Certified therapist with more than 30 years of experience as a speech-language pathologist and teletherapist. She is the owner of S&L Teletherapy Consulting, LLC in De Pere, Wisc. She has been an active participant in ASHA's SIG 18 Telepractice Community and was recently elected to the associate coordinator position within SIG18. She has created multiple online continuing education courses for SLPs considering telepractice. Tracy has contributed articles about speech-language therapy and telepractice, which were featured in *The ASHA Leader*. She frequently presents at state, national, and international levels, having a keen interest in—and commitment to—improving teletherapy services for both the provider and the client.

Do What You Love, Love What You Do

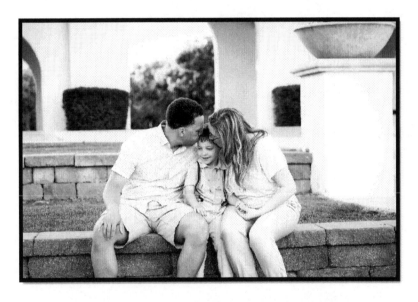

Amy Hill MA, CCC-SLP

Photographer: Brandi Core Photography

* * *

I believe everything happens for a reason, whether you know the reason or not. When I look back on my life and think about the connection of events over time, I am so grateful for each experience as it unfolded.

My dad died the summer before I entered seventh grade, I found my grandmother dead in her home when I was in junior college, I watched my first mother-in-law (one of the most beautiful souls in the world) take her last breath on an Easter morning, and I have been married and divorced twice. Each of these events has brought me strength, resilience, perseverance, and my love for life.

Before my father passed away, he told me, "Make sure you can always take care of yourself." I believe he knew he might not make it through the night, and he needed me to know I could do anything, and I didn't need to rely on others.

At 11 years old, I wasn't able to understand why he said it or what he meant, and I never told anyone about it while I was growing up. I didn't fully understand his intention until I was in graduate school and went through my first divorce. How did I survive those four semesters in graduate school, driving an hour and a half each way to class, working as many hours as I could at the local pharmacy, and trying to figure out how to live on my own? Drive and determination to take care of *me*. No matter where my path would lead me, I was strong, I was determined, and I would take care of myself.

My biggest personal challenge has always been that I am consistently busy, always thinking of ideas and ways to make things more efficient and organized or a little easier for other people. No matter what project, caseload, district, or assignment, I am always learning and changing, updating, and making it easier in some way.

When I was asked to write this chapter, I thought, "Why? Who would want to read what I have to say?"

When I look in the mirror, I see a modest person, a speech-language pathologist (SLP), a mom, and a partner. I have never viewed myself as a *leader,* but I recognize my path has made me a leader. I'm a female leader, a previous small business owner, an association past president, and an instructor. I naturally want to help others, be a sounding board, brainstorm ideas, support others, facilitate learning and continue my own personal and professional development. I am empathetic and genuine. I have a lot of emotions, and the events in the world impact me; they make my heart hurt for those who have lost others, those in pain, and those discriminated against.

Every step leads you to the next step, constantly moving forward, backward, sideways, and eventually forward again. That's what I've come to understand in my nearly 50 years on this planet.

While attending community college in my hometown, Sterling, Colo., I thought I was going to be a teacher and run a developmental child care center. Once I transferred to the University of Northern Colorado, I completed my psychology bachelor degree and chucked my ideas of being a teacher to the wind. To fill my schedule and stay in full-time status, I enrolled in introduction to human communication disorders and sign language classes so I could keep my financial aid. I knew within the first week of these classes that I was going to become an SLP. I could make my love for teaching others specific to communication. I worked hard to take leveling courses, finish my psychology bachelor's degree, and apply to graduate school.

At the end of graduate school, my boyfriend (and later husband) took a job in Arizona, and I went with him. I took the first school placement I found and finished my graduate school placement. I completed my externship and was hired into the district as a school-based SLP.

During my second year, as more families moved to Arizona, my caseload skyrocketed from 65 to nearly 120, and the students ranged from preschool to 8th grade students. I had a speech-language pathology assistant (SLPA), a few middle school teaching assistants who helped me prep materials, an awesome special education team, and an amazing principal. I learned so much during that year about myself, my ability to multitask and organize, and how to work with others while staying focused on my constant "to-do" list.

When I interviewed for my next SLP position, I volunteered to be the lead for the district; the previous person was out on a leave of absence and not returning. I thought, "This is my chance to be a resource for new SLPs, and to make a difference so other SLPs wouldn't feel the way I did during my first three years."

As a lead SLP, I learned how public-school districts work, who makes decisions, and how difficult it is to make long-lasting change. Constant changes in leadership from principals, special education directors, and superintendents all slow the process of creating the ideal school-based SLP position. I grew frustrated because I knew what we needed to do to recruit and retain good staff, but it didn't seem like anyone was listening to me. The priority of a handful of speech staff pales in comparison to the priority of hundreds of new teachers and an economic growth bubble influencing a district's needs.

Professionally speaking, this led to a pivotal period of growth for me. Between 2004 and 2006, I found myself doing three different "jobs." They were sources of inspiration and helped me develop into who I am today: starting a company, becoming president of the Arizona Speech and Hearing Association, and working with Estrella Mountain Community College to start a Speech-Language Pathology Assistant (SLPA) program.

Around this time, a new dream took form. With three other colleagues, I started a school-based contract company where our employees could work in the schools and have the benefits offered by a private company. Using my previous district SLP lead experience, I turned the frustration into a quest for discovering how I could support, mentor, supervise, and be there for people without the added stress of a full-time caseload. Therapists, Educators, Administrators as Mentors in Education (TEAM Ed) was born.

We started by contracting ourselves into schools, and, gradually, hired employees so we could scale back our billable time and increase our level of support. It was difficult, exhausting work, and we worked countless hours. There was no such thing as a 40-hour workweek; it was always 50–60 hours year-round, day in and day out. I didn't realize how much time it takes to be in all departments at once—human resources, payroll, benefits, purchasing, accounts payable and receivable, billing, hiring and recruitment, marketing, professional development, and employee support!

I felt fortunate to have the best three business partners a person could have; we each had our own strengths and focus areas and were all so dedicated. Our employees made more than we did, but we loved what we did, and we kept expanding to cover the overhead.

In time, we grew to about 60 employees, and many decisions were made with our employees' interests in mind, such as offering the best insurance plans we could afford. When difficulties hit our employees, we felt their pain and tried to keep them motivated. We supported employees so they could do the hard job of working with children and families in schools, and then expanded to include early intervention and home-based therapy settings. Coffee shops and restaurants around the state of Arizona became our offices. We searched for small business-friendly banks willing to loan us money with our only collateral being our homes.

We had grown from a couple of client districts and one employee to many client districts and families all over the state. So many times, I sat in my home office thinking about which decision was best for everyone. So many sleepless nights, I wondered how someone would feel because of our decision and if there was enough money in the bank to make payroll and pay expenses. Would I have to go without pay so someone else could feed their family and pay their mortgage?

Although our ownership changed throughout the years, for me, it was never about the money and always about the dream. I was proud of the dedicated employees who accomplished their dreams and also proud to be part of their lives–weddings, divorces, separations, births, out-of-state moves. This overshadowed any negative aspects over the years. I learned how to keep my head high when an employee did something that lost us a district client, when someone didn't show up to work or called out sick too many times, when people did things in their personal lives that impacted their careers, and when I realized how all of the actions of our contracted employees reflected back on the company. Still, we kept moving forward, continuing to be mentors and support our staff. Finding the positive in the negative was a part of who I became.

In 2013, I had to make the most difficult decision of my entire life. My business partner and I were out of money, unable to secure more loans, and the state of Arizona struggled to pay providers under their new early intervention model. We exhausted every funding source and owed hundreds of thousands of dollars to the bank without enough income coming in to cover expenses. We laid off eleven therapists and stopped our home-based therapy business. We weren't alone; other companies around the state also closed during this dark time. Looking my employees, my colleagues, my friends in the eyes and taking their jobs away overnight impacted me at a level I will never forget. I felt guilty about not being able to save some of these jobs, but, in the end, even if I had more money, it wouldn't have been enough. Even writing this now, years later, made me cry, remembering the pain I inflicted on their lives.

During this time, I was pregnant with a miracle little boy, the boy who saved me. He was planned and conceived through in vitro fertilization. When I was going through my medical procedures, I didn't realize how bad things would get. In the last three years of TEAM Ed, I spent all of my personal savings on a horrible second divorce and on trying to conceive my miracle.

Over the next few months, we were barely making ends meet with our school therapists and knew we had to shut it all down. Then, came the second miracle of my year, of my life. A national company found us and admired our passion. Our vision and mission matched what this large corporation wanted to create. Our dream could continue without the stress of owning it.

By the end of that school year, I had my beautiful baby, Sidney, and I took off work for the first time in my life for maternity leave. We also merged our school-based contract company with Learn It Systems. As much as I enjoyed being a small business owner, I was ready to work for someone else. My perspective had changed, and I wanted to focus on myself and my family.

I filed for bankruptcy for the debt incurred and owed the bank for the early intervention home therapy side of the company. Still, it was time for a fresh start, and I was excited to see how I could continue to mentor, supervise, and provide training to therapists. This was the part I loved about my job, and now I could focus on doing all of the things that brought me joy.

I can't tell the story of how I became a leader without including my second inspiration—my passion for supporting Arizona's speech and hearing community.

Around the same time we created TEAM Ed, I jumped headfirst into the Arizona Speech-Language Hearing Association. Since 2004, I have been president-elect, president, past president, CE administrator, state education advocacy leader (SEAL), convention chair, and a variety of committee chairs.

As I was learning how to be a business owner, I also learned to watch, listen, and ask questions. I saw how important gut instincts could be. In 2006, something just didn't feel right. Questions led to bizarre responses which led to more questions, and soon our office administrative secretary confessed to embezzlement. The executive board spent the next decade crawling out of a giant hole, and I had to learn and understand what a fraud investigation entailed. Even in those difficult times, I met even more amazing colleagues who trudged forward in repairing the damage and had *big shoulders* to manage the negative press and the courage to make the association stronger and better.

Over the years, there has not been an issue regarding speech and audiology that I haven't been a part of. I was a part of initial licensing for speech-language pathology assistants, license changes for audiologists, and ongoing legislative efforts to support our field and community.

After my son was born in 2014, I had to step away from something. I chose not to run for any additional executive board positions and, instead, find a better work-life balance. The association will always have a place in my heart, but it is nice to not be in the trenches of the executive board anymore and only participate in committees.

Finally, my story circles to the third and probably most impactful inspiration of my adult life.

Around 2005, I replied to an ad for an SLP at Estrella Mountain Community College. I had no idea what I was getting into: Take a program out of moratorium, teach college classes, create curriculum, and convert curriculum to online classes. WOW! What a learning curve!

I worked with the college to recruit a group of SLPs and became adjunct faculty. For nearly a year, my program team and I spent our evenings eating pizza and writing curriculum, and I led this group through the development of an SLPA program and creation of an online curriculum during a time when online education wasn't yet a popular modality.

As my role at the college expanded and evolved over the past 18 years, I've come to understand adult learners on a whole different level. As such, we made significant improvements in online instruction and in supporting adults, and by interacting with other professors of education, culinary arts, criminal justice, energy, English, economics, science, math, nursing, and anthropology, I have learned even more about working with other people in groups, on committees, and on projects. I have been reminded how a diverse group of people can do anything when they set their minds to it.

Being able to collaborate online, integrate new technologies, collect data on outcomes, and understand the education system from the higher education perspective has helped make me a leader. I love that I am able to impact the lives of so many individuals, who, in turn, impact the education of our speech-language students and clients around the country.

I am proud of my life and what I have accomplished and even though I don't always think of myself as a leader, I lead. Whether I am talking to a new business owner, a new therapist, a seasoned therapist, a professor, a parent, a friend, or a professional, I want to share some little tidbit that helps them in some way. Whether that means thinking about something differently, trying out a new idea, or just filing what I say to maybe use later, it is all about being a mentor.

My passion for speech-language pathology, special education, teaching, and learning has long allowed me to do what I love and, still, love what I do.

Recommendations

If you have an idea, take the risk to run with it as it could be the most wonderful experience of your life. To put it simply:

1. Take risks.
2. Believe in yourself.
3. Build your network of people.
4. Find your passion.

My Wish for You

My wish for you is to be bold, be fierce, and step out of your comfort zone to show your passion to others. Let them see your light!

When we started TEAM Ed, the quote we put on our materials was "do what you love, love what you do." This quote guided us through the ups and downs and continues to be what guides me. Let it be a guide for you. Do what you love, love what you do!

My Community

Watch my interview with Mai Ling Chan on YouTube:

https://bit.ly/amy_hill

Mouse over the QR code with your phone's photo app open to go directly to the interview.

Ways to Connect with Me

Email: amyhill1227@gmail.com

Linked In: https://www.linkedin.com/in/amy-hill-6580a81a/

Facebook: https://www.facebook.com/amysidll

Instagram: @amysid2

Pinterest: Amy Hill

Padlet: amyhill2

Amy Hill is an SLP mentor through and through. For the past two decades, she has owned and sold a company, supervised/mentored a large number of therapists and assistants, supported state legislative issues within the field, created curriculum, and taught many of Arizona's SLPAs.

Silencing the Doubt and Accepting Invitations

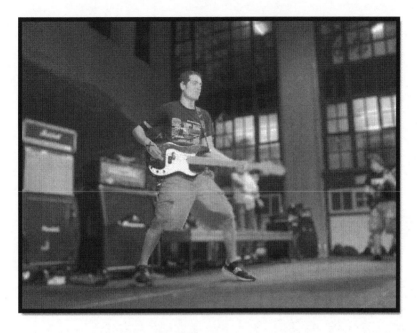

Erik X. Raj, PhD, CCC-SLP

Photographer: Natalie Dallavalle

* * *

From a young age, I appreciated and valued the beauty of communication and, in particular, music.

Music always spoke to me in a riveting way because I believe it is one of the most powerful forms of communication. This is why in 1997, as a shy 13-year-old in middle school who played the bass guitar, I nervously accepted an invitation from my childhood best friends to start a rock band with them. Even though I was petrified of performing in front of others, I still wanted to create and share music with anyone who would listen. Specifically, I wanted to communicate and connect with them through rhythm and song, and thanks to the support and encouragement from my two best friends, I found the courage to do just that.

Between 1998 and 2006, our rock band received the opportunity to leave our home state of New Jersey and tour nationally several times during summer breaks. We played hundreds of concerts, and my wish to connect with thousands of people through rhythm and song not only came true. It gave my life a new direction. This beautiful lived experience of music-based connection was one of the core factors that drove me to study communication sciences and disorders in college and eventually graduate at 24 years old with a master's of science degree in speech-language pathology in 2008. During those wonderful years playing music, I met many people with diverse ways of communicating, and I wanted to know more about those unique qualities. That is exactly what becoming a speech-language pathologist would allow me to do.

A year later in 2009, I was a full-fledged speech-language pathologist working in a school with students ranging from preschool through grade five.

As the saying goes, honesty is the best policy. So, when a fifth grade student on my caseload asked me, "How are you doing today, Mr. Raj?" on this one particular Monday at the start of our therapy session, I sincerely replied, "I'm actually feeling kind of nervous."

I explained to the young person who stutters that I was recently invited to conduct an upcoming thirty-minute educational presentation to a group of speech-language pathologists about stuttering treatment ideas. He genuinely asked me why I was feeling this way, so I confessed to him that I had never done a presentation quite like that before in front of a group of speech-language pathologists, and because of this fact, I was considering politely declining the invitation.

Curiously, even though I had only been a licensed clinician for one year, I felt that I was becoming a clinically competent speech-language pathologist when it came to the assessment and treatment of stuttering. I consistently read the latest stuttering-related research, frequently attended stuttering-related continuing education events, and regularly met with a mentor who was a board-certified specialist in fluency. But, my mind had a habit of trying to "keep me safe" by telling me things that would force me to second-guess myself and the progression I was making as a speech-language pathologist with a special interest in stuttering.

When I received the invitation to present, my internal dialogue went something like this: "You? This has to be a joke. You are way too inexperienced to be presenting to a group of seasoned speech-language pathologists. Don't do it. You'll embarrass yourself."

With my mind racing on, my heart expanded, full of excitement at the possibility of being able to share some of the stuttering treatment ideas I was exploring daily. The tug of war between my mind and heart became exhausting, and, truthfully, it kept me up for many nights.

This tentativeness felt all too familiar to me. I was essentially reliving the same exact feelings I had as a thirteen-year-old when I was invited to start a rock band. My internal dialogue in the face of that invitation similarly was, "You? This has to be a joke. You are way too inexperienced at the bass guitar to be playing in a band. Don't do it. You'll embarrass yourself." Interestingly, I almost politely declined the band's invitation, too, and my "yes" stemmed directly from the spectacular relationship I had with my best friends.

In life, relationships can make all the difference, and this is especially true in the work I did as a newly minted speech-language pathologist. The fifth-grade student I confided in and I had a wonderful client-clinician relationship built on mutual respect. When he asked me how I was doing that Monday, I knew that he was genuinely wondering because he could sense that something was "off" with me. He could sense my nervousness, and he listened closely to my response to his question. Once I was finished, to my surprise, he echoed words to me that I said to him during our therapy sessions.

He reminded me, "In therapy, you always tell me that one of our main goals is to be able to say what we want, when we want."

My jaw dropped. I intentionally kept quiet because I could see in his eyes that he was on to something. He continued, "Believe in yourself and trust the words that you feel are important because if you think they are important, they certainly are and they deserve to be said."

For the first time in my career, I noticed how a healthy amount of what we discuss in therapy, from a stuttering perspective, can connect to instances that go beyond the lens of stuttering and help not only the client, but also the clinician.

Some of the stuttering-related literature I have consumed in my career directly mentions ways in which clinicians can grow and evolve as therapeutic service providers.

For example, one of my favorite published pieces is a 2001 article by Vivian M. Sheehan and Vivian Sisskin.[6] They discussed the intentional decision, as a clinician, to consider revealing one's own personal fear in an effort to better connect with clients and be of better service to them. Sheehan and Sisskin mentioned that, perhaps, a clinician's intense fear of public speaking might be a somewhat similar feeling to what a client who stutters feels sometimes before, during, or after verbally communicating. In sharing that fear-centered information, maybe it could make a positive impact. In my case, I believe that it did.

When I shared my fear about presenting, something transformative occurred. For a few moments, the tables turned and that fifth-grade student was now in the shoes of a clinician, while I took the role of a client. He provided valuable and appropriate words to me so I could get closer to feeling like I could take a chance to face my fear to grow and evolve as a communicator. He politely challenged me to "say what you want, when you want." Regardless of whether I had a communication disorder, this conversation highlighted how our thoughts might very well hold us back, as communicators.

---

[6] Sheehan, Vivian M. and Sisskin, Vivian. "The creative process in avoidance reduction therapy for stuttering." *Perspectives on Fluency and Fluency Disorders* 11.1 (2001): 7-11.

Music also helped bridge what needed to be said in that moment, too.

Believing in the old saying, "Once a musician, always a musician," I always have my acoustic guitar in my therapy room. Though most of my rock star days were already behind me in 2009, that instrument, even now, is the vehicle for playing many tunes and encouraging client-clinician singalongs that connect perfectly to the therapy goals of the students on my caseload. It was true on that Monday, too. Without thinking twice, I picked up the acoustic guitar after receiving the pep talk from that wise fifth grade student, and I started to strum an impromptu song with the following lyrics.

"I owe it to myself,

To say what I want to say.

I owe it to my heart,

To say what I want to say.

I got an invitation,

To share some information.

I got an invitation,

And I'm going to say yes."

The lyrics came right from my heart and were able to easily drown out my mind's unhelpful "don't do it" internal dialogue. The fifth-grade student was bobbing his head to the rhythm of my song, and after the last strum, he stood up and clapped.

"Great job, Mr. Raj," he cheered. He added, "I think you know what your homework assignment is for tonight." I did. It was to accept the invitation.

Several weeks later, I finished the 30-minute educational presentation. I said exactly what I wanted to say to that group of speech-language pathologists. I wanted to communicate and connect with them about the subject of stuttering treatment ideas, and thanks to the support and encouragement of that fifth-grade student, I found the courage to accomplish just that. The encouragement from that youngster forever changed my life, and it has taken me to places I could have never imagined, even in my wildest dreams.

Since beginning my journey as a speech-language pathologist, my special interest in stuttering has always been my guiding light. I believe that when you discover something that magically excites you in ways that are difficult to describe, it is vital to listen to that something and let it take you where it wants to.

As a listener, I was fortunate to hear the knocks of opportunity when, in 2011, I was invited to apply to a doctoral program in communication sciences and disorders, with a concentration in stuttering. I accepted the invitation and, to my surprise, that same year, I was accepted. This newly presented adventure would take me away about 600 miles from New Jersey to Michigan. I packed my car up with as many of my belongings as I possibly could and drove west to officially start my new life as a Detroit-based doctoral student and speech-language pathologist.

One of the things that, sadly, I was unable to bring with me was my acoustic guitar. No matter how I organized the mountains of moving boxes in my car, there was no room for the instrument that I adored. It just would not fit. This bummer of a situation led me to think about technology and how I might be able to still create music in Detroit, but in a slightly different way. One week after moving into my studio apartment in Midtown, I ordered an iPad to quench my music-making thirst.

In 2010, one year before moving to Detroit, Apple Inc. released the first-generation iPad, an exciting tablet computer that some clinicians started to use during the assessment and treatment of various speech-language disorders. The iPad gives users access to the App Store, an online digital distribution platform where individuals can purchase and download digital software applications. Apps, an abbreviation of the word "applications," are software tools that provide additional use and functionality to an iPad, and for myself, I was most interested in apps that would help me create music.

I became an instant fan of the GarageBand app because I did not need my acoustic guitar to use it to unlock its music-making potential. It allowed me to create loads of music thanks to its library of pre-made loops and settings where I was able to play an array of various instruments, digitally, right from within the app.

As an adult, I found this app inspiring, so I could not help but think about how a child might react to it and interact with it. I instantaneously saw how GarageBand could be infused into the assessment and treatment of stuttering. After introducing it to a few of the new students I was working with, these middle school-aged individuals who stutter and I were all hooked in the best possible way.

Like me, these Detroit youngsters loved music, so we frequently created music and performed songs together during our therapy sessions. Often, the melodies we made were accompanied by lyrics that spoke about the lived experience of stuttering. Some of the lyrics from the minds and hearts of those talented students were:

"This voice of mine, let it shine.

Run and hide? Not this time.

This voice of mine, has a choice.

Loud and proud, I'm coming out.

Hear me shout, hear me out.

This voice of mine, let it shine."

This idea to transform my therapy room into a recording studio and concert venue came to me from the same aforementioned 2001 article by Sheehan and Sisskin where they described a client of theirs who composed a song about stuttering that was titled, "Shame." That young musician who stutters wrote lyrics specifically about dealing with the shame associated with stuttering.

Additionally, Sheehan and Sisskin described an adolescent fluency group in which each member wrote a verse of a rap song expressing their feelings related to listener reactions. Then when the lyrics were fully written, they performed the song together. Taking into consideration what I saw, firsthand, in my own music-centered therapy sessions, I believe it is safe to say that the clients Sheehan and Sisskin described were well on their way to growing and evolving as communicators.

Digital technologies, such as iPads and apps, can open many doors for the clients on our caseloads. After immersing myself in many apps like GarageBand, I found myself often saying out loud, "I wish this app had this one particular feature," and asking, "Wouldn't it be cool if I made an app that did this one particular thing?" These are the types of statements and questions that used to trigger my mind's unhelpful "don't do it" internal dialogue, but not anymore. Ever since the support and encouragement of that one fifth grade student in 2009 who reminded me to "say what we want, when we want," things have been different. In the same way that I should say what I want, when I want, I now also do what I want, when I want.

Starting in 2011, I began to teach myself the ins and outs of app development because I wanted to continue creating memorable digital tools and experiences for the individuals on my caseload so they could keep growing and evolving as communicators. From 2012 through 2021, I have successfully developed more than 25 iPad apps for young people with communication difficulties. A number of those digital creations have a musical or auditory focus to them that encourages the individuals to use their voices in a manner that would most certainly be described as "loud and proud."

Since graduating with my doctor of philosophy degree in communication sciences and disorders in 2015, I have been invited to present on the topics of stuttering therapy and digital technology at dozens of state, national, and international educational events. During these events, I have communicated and connected with thousands of speech-language pathologists, and I am beyond grateful for each one of those interactions.

Borrowing from some of the lyrics that were born during past therapy sessions:

"Regarding my presentations,

I let my voice shine.

I do not run and hide.

Not this time.

I have a choice to use my voice,

Loud and proud."

So, as I conclude this chapter, I ask you, the reader, are you saying everything you want, when you want? Are you accepting invitations to communicate and connect with others about subjects and content that fill your heart with excitement? I hope you are, because your words are important, and they deserve to be said. Do not deprive the world of your rhythm and song.

Recommendations

1. Be honest and authentic with the individuals on your caseload because that will positively impact the client-clinician relationship.
2. Recognize the wisdom that all your clients possess because that could not only help you to grow as a clinician, but also as a human.
3. Step outside of your comfort zone and take communication risks because that will show your clients that you are willing to keep growing and evolving as a communicator.
4. Whenever appropriate, use music in the work you do with your clients because, it is fun and functional, and can work with all ages.

My Wish for You

Remember, there is only one you. In every single thing you do, you do you. Rock on!

My Community

Listen to my interview on the Xceptional Leaders Podcast with Mai Ling Chan:

https://bit.ly/erik_raj

Mouse over the QR code with your phone's photo app open to go directly to the podcast.

Ways to Connect with Me

www.erikxraj.com

Email: contact@erikxraj.com

Instagram: @erikxraj

Twitter: @erikxraj

Erik X. Raj holds a Certificate of Clinical Competence from the American Speech-Language-Hearing Association and is a practicing speech-language pathologist who works with school-age children and adolescents with various communication difficulties. He is currently an associate professor in the Department of Speech-Language Pathology at Monmouth University in West Long Branch, New Jersey, and is also a facilitator at Camp Shout Out, a Michigan-based summer camp for young people who stutter. He earned his doctor of philosophy degree in communication sciences and disorders at Wayne State University in Detroit, Mich., as a Thomas C. Rumble University Graduate Fellowship recipient, with additional support from the Kosciuszko Foundation and the American Speech-Language-Hearing Foundation.

It's Not About Me...

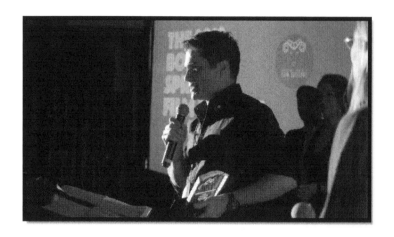

John Gomez, MA, CCC-SLP

* * *

It is surreal to be sitting here again chronicling the journey of my film *WHEN I STUTTER*, adding even more insights about that meaningful, life-changing endeavor.

If you read the prolific Mai Ling Chan's first compendium, *Becoming an Exceptional Leader*, you learned about what inspired the making of that film and some of the challenges I faced. My intent this time is to talk about some of the different ways the documentary has impacted my life, while also revisiting and reinforcing some of the elements I feel will be helpful for anyone on a creative journey.

Making *WHEN I STUTTER* was an experience like no other in my life. It is, by far, the best thing I have done, and I'm so proud of the way that it has influenced the world of stuttering and helped bring much needed awareness to a speech disorder—I like to call it a speech "difference"—that gets very little press. The process of getting the film out to the world was as intensely rich as the experience of making it. People worldwide have come to embrace my film and herald it for being earnest and heartfelt. Along the way, I have made many new connections and friends. These connections are invaluable; they provide meaning like no material object ever could. Not a day goes by where I do not do something on behalf of the film. The duties entail setting up screenings, implementing foreign language subtitles, and responding to emails from those who were touched by the film, among other things. I often liken the distribution of a documentary to raising a child. My child is four years old now and has gained some independence, but, of course, it still needs a parent.

One of the most empowering things we can do is share our vulnerabilities. It's humanizing, demystifying, and it lets people know that they are not alone when they encounter similar obstacles in their lives.

It would be nice to tell you that making *WHEN I STUTTER* was a work of divine inspiration and that it came together with minimal struggle, but that would be untrue. There were many barriers to making the film. Some of the challenges were external, such as securing funding, finding subjects, and capturing the right shots. However, many of the barriers to making the film resided inside of me, and I learned, from talking to other filmmakers and artists, that embarking on any creative endeavor usually entails staring down your inner demons.

Perhaps the most significant challenge was feeling as though I was unworthy of doing such a project. After all, I didn't have any formal training in filmmaking, and my only experience in the medium came from being a wedding videographer. There came a certain point in the project where I had filmed my participants and I knew I had good raw material. But, I also knew the project lacked cohesion. I asked myself questions such as "Should I have mapped it all out before I started?" Or, "Should I have immersed myself in 'how to make a documentary' material before starting?" Perhaps the most pernicious question of them all was, "Should I, John Gomez, have ever dreamt of making this film?"

Self-doubt in creative people is an interesting concept to contemplate—it's almost a contradiction in terms. In place of any professional knowledge, you'll have to settle for my dime-store psychology theory of why self-doubt in creative people is paradoxical.

To say "I am going to make a film" takes a certain amount of nerve and, well, um, a sizable ego. So one must have some delusions of grandeur in attempting such an undertaking. Yet, at the same time, there is a diminishing element in that same person that makes them feel as though they can't properly execute the very project they proclaimed that they could. This begs the question, "Why say that you can make a film if you don't think that you are capable of making said film?" It's contradictory, puzzling.

Exploring why self-doubt exists at all could be fuel for a whole other book. And, while I don't understand the paradox fully, I know what gets you through self-doubt. At least, I know what got me through those rough patches. I remembered why I embarked on this journey in the first place. The answer was simple: It was never about me.

My inspiration to finish the film came largely from the people who contributed to the film's creation as participants and co-creators. It also came from friends lending their time and talent to the endeavor.

Without the candor and raw vulnerability from the interviewees, there is no *WHEN I STUTTER,* or at least not one that is honest. No amount of flashy production value or star power could ever supersede the power of the truth. Hearing about the reality of how stuttering impacts the whole person was also inspirational, like rocket fuel.

Inspiration also went hand-in-hand with responsibility. There was a responsibility "to get it right" so the words of the participants would reverberate powerfully to the audience. To this day, the film often brings audience members to tears. I don't think the tears entirely arise because of sadness or sympathy for the participants; rather, it is because people can relate to some of the humanistic elements of stuttering even if they don't stutter themselves. Feelings of isolation and being "the outsider" don't solely exist in people who stutter; they are part of the human condition.

Audiences also relate to uplifting themes such as the powerful release that comes from significant—sometimes life-saving—emotional breakthroughs. Relating to these elements allows audience members to build bridges from their life experiences to those of the film's participants.

The life experiences that the participants revealed not only made for a revelatory film, but it has also revolutionized the way I think as an SLP (speech-language pathologist). Effectively treating adults who stutter isn't about remediating a set of isolated behaviors to make them fluent. It's about treating the whole person and acknowledging that they are on an important journey toward self-discovery. With this philosophy, I am more of a counselor that helps my clients find what it is about their communication that they want to explore. What do they care about? What do they fear? What are their strengths? Who are they, beyond their stuttering? What do they see as their ultimate goal? Again, it's not about me. Stuttering treatment is most effective when it focuses on a client's values.

As a school-based speech pathologist, I occasionally have the pleasure of working with a child who stutters. Stuttering is a low-incidence communication disorder, with only 1% of the population comprised of people who stutter.[7] Therefore, a student who stutters does not often pop up on your caseload as often as those with, say, articulation or expressive language concerns. Nonetheless, I know that this child is at a critical juncture in their development as a communicator.

When I work with a child who stutters, I am often reminded of what has been imparted to me by so many adults who stutter. Namely, that speech therapy itself had been a detriment to them instead of a benefit. This is because so much of mainstream stuttering therapy focuses on making children fluent. The act of stopping and redirecting a child every time they stutter can build a vicious inner critic within that child. That inner critic will often grow and grow because they have come to see their stuttering as a "bad thing," and

---

[7] FAQ. Stuttering Foundation: A Nonprofit Organization Helping Those Who Stutter. (n.d.). Retrieved September 19, 2021, from https://www.stutteringhelp.org/faq.

every time it happens, they think that they must fight against it or avoid it. As a result, their stuttering can become much more severe later in life.

You may ask, why does stuttering get worse under these conditions? The baseline organic stuttering a person had as a child may have been classified as "mild." However, in trying to fight or avoid those moments of stuttering, muscular tension and a whole host of unneeded behaviors can develop. These factors can make the act of stuttering more difficult and severe over time. Knowing that stuttering can worsen because of what I do as a therapist is a consequence I always have in mind when working with children who stutter.

Ultimately, my therapy aims to have the child build confidence so they "say what they want, when they want, whether or not they stutter." This is not a concept I came up with on my own. I heard this idea from Dr. Dale Williams, who is a participant in *WHEN I STUTTER*. I love this quote, and it has become my mantra for stuttering therapy.

When you break the quote down, it disregards fluent speech and emphasizes confidence, assertiveness, and the bigger picture of communication itself. Everything I do in therapy with children who stutter is an attempt to make them robust communicators, whether they stutter or not. I preach this approach to therapy far and wide now that I have a platform to do so.

Shortly after releasing the film, I was offered a teaching position at my alma mater, California State University, Los Angeles. The department head and my former professor, Dr. Cari Flint, reached out to me and asked me if I'd like to teach the graduate-level stuttering course. I was beyond flattered, and while I was unsure of my ability to teach at that level, I accepted the challenge.

Four years later, I find myself teaching several courses at Cal State LA and loving every minute of it. I now get to influence future SLPs and impart these humanistic themes that surround communication disorders in the best way that I can. This opportunity alone has been such a privilege and added a dimension to my life that is irreplaceable.

I have also made some great friendships along the way. I recently heard a statistic about the average male not having even one person they can truly refer to as a friend. If that truly is the case, then I am an aberration because I have several wonderful friends. The kind who make life worth living . . . the kind who support you . . . the kind who let you know they have your back no matter what! Some of these beautiful souls I knew before the film; they were instrumental in helping me make it. Some friends I made during the making of the film and throughout the distribution process. They are equally precious to me.

I also feel fortunate that *WHEN I STUTTER* has managed to make a profit. In meeting and talking with documentary filmmakers across the world, I realize that this is a rarity. Most documentary films do not make back their budget, let alone turn a profit. My documentary has sustained itself primarily because of educational sales to over 100 universities and organizations worldwide. My film is being used to educate hearts and minds globally, and this was always my greatest hope for the film.

The last thing I would like to share is a carbon copy from *Becoming an Exceptional Leader.* I am quoting this portion because I believe that this quality has helped me more than any other in my life's journey. With a clear conscience, I cannot avoid talking about the central role of resilience in my life.

If I have a gift, I would have to say that it is one that I share with a fictitious boxing character from Philadelphia who came to the world's attention in 1976, Rocky Balboa. I have always loved the idea of Rocky because he represents such a gritty and heartfelt version of the American Dream. The interesting part is that he wasn't a great fighter in the classical sense. Instead, his boxing abilities were depicted as crude and underwhelming. He did have one great gift: He could withstand more punishment than the next guy. In his fights, Rocky would get knocked down only to get back up time after time. One time his manager even urged him to "stay down" for safety reasons, but he just got back up again. In the end, he was able to take more punches than his opponent, and he was literally the last man standing.

This is where we overlap. I feel that resilience is my gift, too. Although I probably couldn't take a lot of real punches, not like Rocky anyway, I do have a high threshold for pain, disappointment, and all manner of setbacks that life can throw at me. It may be inadvisable at times, but I keep getting back up and moving forward. It's a necessity.

Recommendations

1. **Surround yourself with positive and honest people.** Any meaningful endeavor will be fraught with self-doubt, and you don't need negativity from people further hampering your project. Having the right people around you will make all the difference—trust me.

Nothing will kill a project like negativity and the constant sowing of doubt. On the other end of the spectrum, having people tell you that something is "great" when it's not is also not productive. A balance can be struck between positivity and honesty. They need to go hand-in-hand for a project to grow.

2. **Choose your medium for sharing your story.** If you are going into filmmaking, know that you have picked one of the most challenging ways to express your artistic or educational vision. While no path is ever "easy," other avenues might be more fitting. An outlet such as writing is less taxing and much less expensive, and so are many other creative options. If a story can be effectively told in any other way, for example, as an article, a book, a blog, a podcast, through photography, then I'd highly recommend telling it that way. But if it MUST be conveyed visually through a film, know that many challenges lie ahead. Be resilient—KEEP GOING!

3. **Set a deadline.** Set goals for yourself to present your material (even rough versions of it) at specific points in time. At least for me, deadlines can be very galvanizing for a project. While this may put some time pressure on you, it will keep you focused on a specific point in time when you will be asked to put forth something presentable. It may not be representative of your best work or even the final product, but it will keep you moving forward. Sometimes the quest for perfection can stifle a project. A less-than-perfect idea that has been put into the world is far better than a perfect idea that will never be shared. I believe this to be true in

education as well as art. Leonardo da Vinci is believed to have said, "Art is never finished, only abandoned." What if he had never shared his work because it wasn't perfect?

My Wish for You

As any director will tell you, setbacks can and will occur when making a film. Sometimes they are devastating. You just have to get up and keep moving forward. Successfully contending with the setbacks I faced when making *WHEN I STUTTER* has only reinforced my belief in the essential nature of resilience in an artist's life. Resilience may be one of the greatest assets we can have when taking on a big project.

In your creative endeavors, my wish for you is to "GET UP" every time you feel knocked down. Count on setbacks because they will always be there! There will be self-doubt, naysayers, financial difficulty, lapses in judgment, a lack of confidence, a feeling of being lost, and on and on. Get up, and move forward!

My Community

Listen to my episode on the Xceptional Leaders podcast:

https://bit.ly/john_gomez

Mouse over the QR code with your phone's photo app open to go directly to the podcast.

Ways to Connect with Me

Website:
www.WhenIStutter.org

Email: john@whenistutter.org

Facebook: When I Stutter

Instagram: @when_i_stutter

IMDB: When I Stutter

John Gomez works as a speech pathologist for the Los Angeles Unified School District and as a professor at California State University, Los Angeles. He is also a documentary filmmaker. His feature film, *WHEN I STUTTER*, has been in more than 16 film festivals worldwide and has won seven awards. John was honored with the Lois V. Douglass Distinguished Alumnus Award from CSULA and the Emerging Filmmaker Award from the Chagrin Documentary Film Festival.

Can't Fail

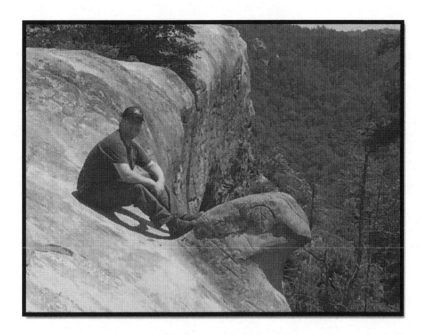

Matthew Hott MA, CCC-SLP

* * *

The biggest challenge in the creation of the Speech Science podcast was me.

Besides being my own biggest critic and enemy to the creative process, I came from a radio, television, and theater background where there is always a fine line of how information and art are consumed and valued.

In the radio and television news world, it's all about how quickly you can get the information out there with the nicest packaging. But it does not live forever. Once it's consumed, very rarely does it live on.

The same is true with live theater. You can attend a show multiple times, and each time something is different. An actor may take a new risk one night that results in the greatest performance ever seen on stage. Or the risk may be a failure, and becomes his or her worst performance. Either way, each night is different, and the fleeting moment of that performance doesn't last to be seen by others over and over.

But I have also worked on projects that were designed to be consumed many times. With these projects, there is a tendency to become so involved in fixing one small detail that you lose track of time. Perfection becomes the focus.

So in creating a weekly or bi-weekly podcast, I've had to marry both the "consume and forget" culture of news and the need for perfecting a product that can be consumed and appreciated multiple times, over and over again.

I see now how these complementary opposites have unfolded for me over the course of my life and with the help of others who showed up along the way.

Some of it started in college, at Muskingum College (now Muskingum University), where as an undergraduate I studied communications with a focus on digital media convergence (the blending of radio, television, theater, and print journalism).

Jerry Martin, a Ph.D. better known as "Doc Martin," was my theater professor and my academic advisor at Muskingum University. He would always say (I'm not sure to this day if he was joking or not), "Never let details get in the way of a good story."

In my junior year, we saw him create a show for no other reason than to create a show. He would appreciate that I don't remember all of the details, but the story is still a good one. I watched him revise and perfect his show on a made-up conversation between Mark Twain and Teddy Roosevelt. Through this process, I was able to learn how to get an audience to care about what you are doing. The key to this was to care about it yourself. If you cared about it, then the audience would buy-in.

After college, I worked at a local television station in Ohio. One of my first bosses was Brian Wagner. I worked for him at WHIZ, where I was the play-by-play guy for high school football and a director for the nightly newscast. I learned from him and his philosophy, "Say whatever you want, but believe what you say." For me, this meant that I could have an opinion as long as I believed my opinion, something that would follow me forward all the way through my media and theater career, through my shift toward speech-language pathology, and into the podcasting world.

Another pivotal moment came a few years later when I was working at WETM, the local NBC affiliate, and Backyard Broadcasting, a radio cluster in Elmira, a small city in upstate New York. While at WETM, I worked with anchor Naveen Dhaliwal, who is now at ABC7 in New York. In between shows, she told me she was a part-time SLP (speech-language pathologist) and worked with children on her days off.

This sparked my curiosity, and I began researching SLP. The more I read, the more I wanted to learn about the field and the entrance requirements. I just did not know if I was ready to leave my media and theater work and start in a new direction.

Life, as it sometimes does, helped me make the choice.

In the winter of 2008, I was at an all-time low on the enjoyment factor in my job. I felt I was not pursuing anything of value. I had told myself years before when I left St. Xavier High School in Cincinnati that I would continue to "live the fourth" (living the promises I made on the fourth day of Kairos Jesuit retreat back in 2004), but I wasn't living that promise. I was just doing what I could to get by.

The day after Christmas, after working a 16-hour shift sustained by fast food and frozen dinners, I quit my radio and television career and took a bold leap of faith.

That week, I went to the Arnot Mall in upstate New York, picked out a ring, and then on January 2, 2009, drove more than 10 hours to surprise my girlfriend Kim. I told her I wanted to marry her, take a gamble on leveling courses, and, if I was lucky, go to grad school for speech therapy. She astonished me with a "Yes!" and waited more than two years for our wedding so I could make graduate school a reality.

By the summer of 2009, I was at Kent State University, living in the cheapest apartment I could find and taking the prerequisite classes I needed for graduate school. Afterward, I attended Ohio University, again living in the cheapest apartment I could find, and completed my master's in 2013.

Even though I was embarking on a new path, I still enjoyed aspects of radio, television, and theater. I just didn't want anyone to tell me what to say.

The natural extension of this eventually turned into the Speech Science podcast. I saw it as something that would outlast my time on this earth, and blend the parts of my previous work that I loved with my new career.

As these things sometimes go, Speech Science started with a chance encounter, a conversation, and the spark of an idea that evolved and developed into its current format that hits your iPhone or podcast player 30 times a year.

The chance encounter was meeting Lucas Steuber (you can read his chapter in *Becoming an Exceptional AAC Leader*) at an ASHA (American Speech–Language–Hearing Association) conference in Denver. We kicked it off well, and, later in the day, I met him in a hotel bar for drinks with his wife and my friend, Michelle Wintering, who would become a future co-host. We made some jokes about how we should do a male perspective podcast for speech therapy, but then realized we were severely underselling our scope of content.

A few weeks later, Lucas and I were exchanging phone calls and texts about the show and what it would take to make it happen. Lucas would have a comment or an idea about the business side of it, and I would dig in to start building it out. When the show launched, I became the de facto executive producer, editor, and lead host training Lucas, Ivan Campos, and Chandru Vitale on the first 40 or so episodes.

After completing 144 episodes with more than 2,300 weekly listeners in 12 countries, I will be the first to say that I have gained nothing financially from this show! I pay more to keep my personal enjoyment on-air than anything we have earned over the years.

So what have I *gained* from doing this show?

Personally, my resolve to conquer the world at my own pace has been strengthened. I have also learned that if I set my mind to it, then I can create a show that is listened to by more than 2,000 people a week!

More importantly, though, my sons mirror what I do, and I have fostered a love and enjoyment for them to create something in this world (my daughter, only 11 months old at the time of writing of this, has not shown the urge to create art, just yet!). My boys put on their headsets and create their own podcasts talking about their video games. They don't do it for others to listen. They do it to carve out their own space in the world. That's the greatest thing this podcast has done for me: I have modeled a way for my children to carve their own spaces, and to create their own art.

Essentially, that was the bridge between my media, theater, and SLP careers. I knew I wasn't creating a show solely for the purpose of making others happy. I knew I wanted to create a show that would make me happy. The challenge was to figure out how to do that.

In doing this show, I never set out to become an influencer or to create something others would want to listen to. Instead, I sat down and created a show that married my radio background with my speech knowledge. I wanted to be happy with the end product, and ultimately, that's all I cared about.

What also helped was being able to accept criticism and still remain dedicated to creating the offering I wanted to create.

In theater, radio, and television, I developed a very thick skin. We would pay people and consulting teams to listen to or watch our résumé reel and then critique our skills. We would be told to cut our hair, wear better clothes, quit using filler words, change our speed or our cadence, or even our name.

So when it came time to create the podcast show, I knew I could handle anyone's critiques because the show wasn't for them, it was for me. I spent too many years, and an undergrad degree, pursuing art that made others happy. This show wasn't for others— it was for me. I wanted something I could share with my family. I wanted something that my kids could listen to and hear my voice and my thoughts.

I wish I could sit here and tell you I doubted that we would make it as a show, but that would be false modesty. It's not that I was arrogant about the show, but it couldn't fail because there was no way to measure success or failure. If I was happy with it, it succeeded. If I wasn't happy with it, I changed it to make myself happy. I learned this in high school and remembered it again later in life.

This reminds me of something I heard Kevin Smith say on his podcast. He spoke about how creating a podcast is creating art. He said it didn't matter how many people listened, if it was one person or 1 million people, but what was important was that you created something that no one else can take away, something that will live forever.

In this same podcast, he spoke about how there is no competition in podcasting, that a rising tide raises all boats. That's what made me want to create the Speech Science show and do it for myself: doing it for myself helps all of us rise. It's very easy to listen to critiques from others not doing it, but if you can learn to ignore the voices from the outside and listen to what makes you happy, then you can create art that you enjoy.

Recommendations

I am not the person to give great advice on how to succeed because my success was all personal. I challenge those who are doing what they are doing with this question: WHY? Why are you doing this? Who cares about the how or where or how good? It's the WHY.

Once you figure out your why, then I recommend you do it for those reasons. Is it to make money, make yourself happy, to get free stuff? If you set out and create your own answer to the question WHY, then you have determined your success or failure.

My WHY was because I wanted to talk on the radio again but didn't want anyone to tell me what to talk about. I wanted my kids, wife, and family to hear it and say, "Oh cool he's doing that."

Do your art to complete the answer to your own WHY question. With that in mind, I recommend—

1. Ask yourself why.
2. Do it to answer the WHY question.
3. Don't let anyone else change your answer.

My Wish for You

My wish for you when you are creating something is that you know that you are special. You are awesome, and you are doing something that no one else can do or take away from you. Who cares how technically good you are at something, how great it looks or sounds. This doesn't mean anything. What does mean something is that you are taking the time to share your abilities, your view, your inspiration with the world. You are giving the world a gift. It doesn't matter if it's drawn, or spoken, or filmed, or signed. You have added to the history of this planet by adding your own thing to it that no one can take away. Do it for as long as you want to; then stop. Come back to it later. But just know that you have created something that no one else could do or has done or will ever do.

My Community

Listen to my interview on the Xceptional Leaders Podcast with Mai Ling Chan:

https://bit.ly/matt_hott

Mouse over the QR code with your phone's photo app open to go directly to the podcast.

Ways to Connect with Me

@matthewhott

m-hott@hotmail.com.

www.speechsciencepodcast.com

Matt Hott graduated from Muskingum University in 2007 with a degree in communications and with a master's in speech and language pathology from Ohio University in 2013. He lives in Cincinnati with his wife (Kim) and their three children (Michael, Andrew, and Evelynn). Matt has served as the Ohio Speech-Language-Hearing Association's school representative and the Ohio ASHA SEAL (state education advocacy leader) from 2015–2016 and 2017–2021.

When Minorities Unite, We Become the Majority

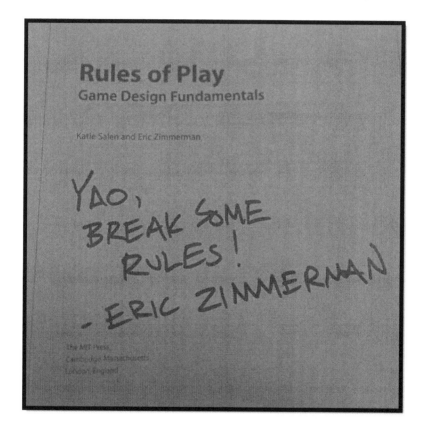

Yao Du, PhD, CCC-SLP

* * *

I pride myself in having two identities: a bilingual Mandarin-English speaking speech-language pathologist (SLP), and human-computer interaction (HCI) researcher who designs and evaluates technology for individuals with communication impairments. These two identities have offered me unique perspectives to not only serve culturally and linguistically diverse clients but also share the same discourse with technology designers and developers.

As a first-generation immigrant in the United States, I consider my story of developing these two identities as one of the many minority voices that can grow louder if we unite.

My family has a long history of communication impairments. My father was a stutterer, my grandmother suffered from a right hemisphere stroke, and I have personally experienced the behavioral, emotional, and social challenges of living in a family with individuals with disabilities. Neither my father nor my grandmother received speech therapy due to a lack of resources and care in China. To date, in China, there is still no uniform organization that systematically regulates and offers training resources in the same way as the American Speech-Language-Hearing Association (ASHA).

After moving to the United States at age 16 with my family, I overcame multiple socioeconomic and cultural-linguistic barriers and became a first-generation college student. Like many other students, I worked different part-time jobs to support my family and supply my living expenses. Although some of these initial jobs (such as cashier at karaoke bars, insurance call representative, and behavioral coach for adult day programs) paid a minimum wage, I was later able to leverage these unique opportunities in Silicon Valley and made connections that helped me find work at many startup companies in the educational and health space. Two years after receiving my license, to alleviate my family and my financial burdens, I was able to pay off all my student loans before going back to school for my doctoral degree. It was also from these part-time jobs that I learned to develop non-clinical skills, including customer service, teaching, and technology proficiency, which eventually became instrumental to my future career development.

My understanding of my minority identity was relatively naïve until the first awakening moment in my undergraduate child psychology class taught by Dr. A, a Hispanic male with a clinical doctorate. My favorite part of this class was watching Dr. A engage in a brutal self-reflection intertwined with his life story, his race and ethnicity, and scientific research.

When discussing the interdisciplinary research across psychology and neuroscience, Dr. A pointed to his brain and said, "Here, my amygdala stores all the memories with my Caucasian ex-girlfriend. I was prepared to spend the rest of my life with her, but her parents did not accept my Hispanic descent. Such trauma existed in psychology and also in neuroscience."

When discussing research bias in his field, Dr. A was frankly honest, "In my clinical psychology doctoral program, I was the only Hispanic student in my cohort. When I read about all the papers published by white Caucasian scholars, all I want to do is shout to my professor, 'Bull shit! Growing up as a Hispanic male child, I have a say on this. What's stated in this research study is NOT true!'"

It was the first course where I heard personal stories about race from a clinically licensed minority faculty member at a teaching university. Many years later, I learned about qualitative research and read about the power of storytelling as a doctoral student; I myself also became a minority faculty member in speech-language pathology at a teaching university in the middle of the Covid-19 global pandemic and the climax of the "Stop Asian Hate" Movement. I realized that throughout my professional career, many minority faculty members such as Dr. A spoke their individual narratives as counter-stories against systemic racism, and their past stories have become the prelude of my story right now.

Motivated to help individuals with communication disorders, I completed two degrees—a bachelor's degree at San Jose State University and a master's degree at the University of Texas, Austin. Being one of the few students in my program who did not grow up speaking English, I used my non-native language to assess and treat clients, teach undergraduates, serve in student leadership roles, and complete a master's thesis on bilingual Mandarin-English language assessment morphosyntax test development.

Although both institutions are filled with diverse student populations and are located in linguistically diverse cities like San Jose, California, and Austin, Texas, I have always been the only student from mainland China in my cohort. Even during my clinical fellowship year and later years as a licensed SLP in California, I was often the only bilingual SLP in my clinical environment. I have been mocked about my accent which did not impact my intelligibility, and I have been judged as "not competent" by family members who do not want to be treated by a non-white clinician.

However, I did not let my unique identity become a barrier to become a better clinician, and instead, I used my bilingual skills to advance the access of care to people who share the same cultural and linguistic backgrounds as me. Working with clients as young as 18 months and as old as 108 years, I was able to provide consultation and parent coaching to Mandarin-speaking children with suspected stuttering at private clinics, interpret for caregivers and other medical staff members at my hospital for adults who acquired a brain injury due to a fall at home, and also implement old pop songs from a Taiwanese singer during melodic intonation therapy with patients with aphasia at my skilled nursing facility.

On one hand, it has been extremely rewarding to help these individuals with communication disorders become better communicators; on the other hand, I witnessed emerging technologies' limitation in socio-technical design that has impacted usability, access, and equity. For example, while children with complex communication needs benefited from assistive technology applications such as augmentative and alternative communication (AAC) systems; poor usability and increased technology abandonment have failed to meet many parents' expectations.

Also, while clinicians have benefited from computer-based electronic medical records (EMRs), EMRs have been increasingly adopted as workplace applications on mobile tablets, leading to ridiculous documentation expectations and work productivity at some facilities. This means, after being given an iPad loaded with an EMR software, I was expected to complete my clinical notes while directly treating patients to minimize non-direct treatment time. These industry practices challenged me to rethink ethical practice at the workplace, and as I became dissatisfied with my monthly salary, I couldn't stop asking myself: What if I could share my vision about how to create the technology and make the workplace better with all the people involved in the healthcare ecosystem—the health professionals and their patients, as well as individuals who build the health and assistive technology?

Inspired by the vision to improve the quality and governance of health and assistive technology, I decided to go back to school for a full-time doctoral degree in informatics at the University of California, Irvine (UCI). My doctoral research projects were directly drawn from my clinical experience working with children with communication impairments (CwCI) in educational and medical settings. During my doctoral years, I gained technical knowledge and training to design, evaluate, and implement various web, mobile, and voice interfaces for CwCI and their key stakeholders (such as parents, SLPs, mobile app designers, and developers).

As a woman in the field of computing who has a clinical background, I have encountered several challenges during my first year in my graduate program. Because my research topics are at the forefront of innovation, connecting multiple disciplines and areas of research (including digital health, digital literacy, and assistive technology), initially I struggled to find faculty advisors and committee members with shared research interests and background knowledge to support my work. This requires me to expand my research network and develop an understanding of different epistemological beliefs outside my clinical domain as an SLP.

Another challenge is the shortage of specific funding in this interdisciplinary area of research. Existing academic and industry research funding in computing typically emphasizes STEM-related subjects and not in special education technology. Studying at a non-clinical program has limited my opportunity to receive specific clinical grants because many grants only support students in traditional clinical research programs. These struggles led to an extremely difficult first year in my doctoral program, but I had my breakthrough when I redirected my attention to invest in the growth and development of my undergraduate students.

During the four years of my doctoral program, I have mentored seven graduate students in SLP and led independent studies and capstone projects for three cohorts of more than 20 UCI undergraduate students from different majors, such as informatics, public health, and game design. Many students were also first-generation college students like myself. Although they were passionate about designing accessible tools to support children with disabilities, they lacked the opportunity to engage in interdisciplinary research due to the lack of an SLP program in the entire University of California system, which is known for its research but not clinical professional training programs. I used my clinical and technical knowledge to educate my students on digital tools for users with disabilities, and also supported their career development and continued pursuit of graduate degrees. With support from amazing faculty mentors, I taught my students both qualitative research methods such as interview, app store review, and video analysis, as well as quantitative methods like conducting experiments and surveys.

These research experiences allowed me to collaborate with scholars from various geographic locations in the United States, namely California, Delaware, and Texas. Working collaboratively with clinicians, researchers, and developers, I participated in many projects, such as a web-based language assessment tools so parents can administer receptive language assessment to their bilingual children at home, and a voice game that allows young children to speak to the conversational agent Amazon Alexa during a quiz game. Additionally, I also have the opportunity to enrich my industry experiences through internships with a startup company that aims to use machine learning algorithms combined with parent questionnaires and child video analysis to obtain early developmental screening through mobile health applications. These projects have been published and presented at interdisciplinary research communities in game design, medical informatics, and assistive technology, as well as at ASHA.

My two identities, a bilingual Mandarin-English speaking SLP and an HCI researcher, have enabled me to re-examine my contribution to the field of speech-language pathology and create a different mission: Help clinicians better understand how technology is designed, from the perspective of functional requirements, prototyping, design and development, and evaluation, and assist technologists to design better solutions for clinicians as well as their clients.

One of the most important lessons I learned is that when transforming clinical knowledge into creativity, there's an inevitable loss in translation, resulting in probably only 10% of the ambitious vision going into actual production. When I got my first iPad in 2012 and saw how a child with autism leveraged Proloquo2Go to gain his voice, I felt like I was worshiping technology designers and innovators such as Steve Jobs, rather than the intersectionality of the art and technology behind his legend.

Now that I have personally grown to be a clinician innovator, I realize how successful technological design in combination with modern medicine can bring harmony to the field of speech pathology. In one of my data collection sessions at a participant's home, after playing with the app my team built, a 6-year-old boy asked about the virtual avatar who spoke to him: "Is she real?" In that moment, I see his sparkling eyes filled with excitement about the physical and virtual worlds, and this is what I want to build for the next generation of youth with disabilities: Equal opportunities to communicate freely and safely through interactive media and technology.

Recommendations

Speaking from my two identities, I share these personal recommendations with you, especially minority clinicians and researchers, as well as those who are passionate about building better technology for our future generations:

1. Challenge the system by breaking and changing rules.
2. Mentor the next generation to design technology and provide services that assist the users and against abusers.
3. Develop multifaceted identities to engage in interdisciplinary and translational research. It will change your worldview.

My Wish for You

To anyone who speaks English as a second language in this profession: Having an accent could significantly increase the social and communication pressure to second language learners. However, everyone has an accent. It is considered a language difference rather than a disorder. Having an accent means that during communication, one can comprehend and speak at least more than one language or dialect. This should be a strength that people feel proud of, rather than a weakness that brings shame and self-doubt. I hope that all minorities who are confronting systemic racism in this country can unite to share their stories because resistance is our existence.

To anyone who works at the forefront of technology design and development, remember that technology should be designed by the people and for the people. If you are frustrated and complaining or have an innovative idea to share, whether it is no-tech or high-tech, don't waste time merely working for others. Instead, stop complaining and start building. Because if you truly care about something, no one is motivated to make it better except you. Everything will take longer than you might think. We need to let our minds think and move faster than technological advancement.

My Community

Watch my interview with Mai Ling Chan:

https://bit.ly/yao_du

Mouse over the QR code with your phone's photo app open to go directly to the interview.

Ways to Connect with Me

Twitter: @YaoDuSLP

LinkedIn: @YaoDu

Dr. Yao Du is a clinician and design researcher who advocates and creates accessible technology to break through traditional healthcare service delivery for individuals with disabilities.

The Leap From School-Based SLP to the State's Superintendent of Public Instruction

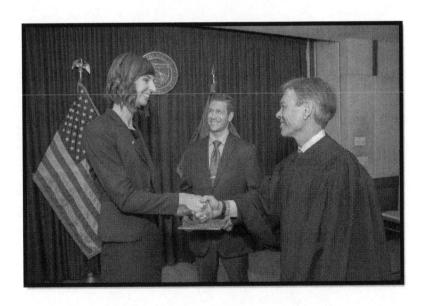

Kathy Hoffman, MS, CCC-SLP

* * *

My first position as a speech-language pathologist was at an elementary school in the Vail School District in Tucson, Ariz. The school overlooked the desert landscape to the east and a suburban housing community to the west. The district

93

proudly offered an inclusive special education program for children with disabilities and attracted many military families who were stationed at the nearby Air Force base.

I met Mason[8] at Vail. He was a first grade student who transferred into my school and was nonverbal due to brain damage from severe epilepsy. Although we say "nonverbal" for students like Mason, he was far from quiet. At the beginning of the school year, Mason was loud, disruptive, and drew a lot of negative attention from the school leaders.

I met with his mother to determine the best mode of communication for him, and she shared that he owned an iPad with the TouchChat app, but it had never worked for him so they relied on picture cards. At home, they used five basic picture cards to meet his needs. I asked for permission to try TouchChat again. His mom agreed.

Although it would have been ideal to seek a new AAC (augmentative and alternative communication) evaluation, Mason's behaviors were disrupting his peers and preventing him from participating in class. Finding a solution quickly became a priority.

I started experimenting with TouchChat to see how functional it would be for him and determined that he was a fast learner. He quickly exceeded my expectations and his vocabulary exploded. His teacher and parents noticed a positive difference in his behaviors and social skills as he found new ways to express himself. I reflected on how Mason had started with only his five picture cards, and how by the

---

[8] The student's name was changed to protect his identity.

end of the school year, he could say his friends' names, request his favorite games, and, most importantly, say "I love you" to his mom.

At school, kids learn much more than academic skills. The speech therapy services that are part of special education programs are critical for developing life skills. As I continued advancing my career, I loved working with students from all backgrounds to make a difference not only in their school experiences, but in their lives.

A few years later, my husband and I moved two hours north from Tucson to Phoenix, and I started a new position at a Title I K-8 school in the Peoria Unified School District. Title I schools receive federal funds to support low-income students throughout the nation, and the impact of the 2008 economic recession on our school grew more evident as Arizona leaders made significant cuts to public education. Nearly a decade after these cuts, I noticed that school resources were still sparse, and the cost of resources was often passed on to educators and families. I started to tune in to education funding policies at the state and federal level to understand why there was such a strain on special education resources and why so many of my colleagues were deciding to leave the teaching profession.

In February 2017, I watched the confirmation hearing of Betsy DeVos, who was nominated as the U.S. Secretary of Education. How could someone who had not worked in a school lead the country's public education system? My stomach turned. My mind raced.

In Arizona, we had a parallel situation at the state level. For more than 20 years, non-educators had been elected to be the superintendent of public instruction and led the Arizona Department of Education. I thought to myself, "We need educators leading in education, people who understand the ins and outs of the schools to inform policy decisions at all levels."

There had never been a moment when I considered changing career paths because I loved working as an SLP (speech-language pathologist) in our schools. However, the next morning, I sat with my husband on our patio eating breakfast and I said, "You're going to think I'm crazy . . ." Within a couple of weeks, I had officially filed to run for superintendent of public instruction.

I was a first-time candidate with no political connections, a young woman, 31 years old, and fearless enough to run for state office. I had never run for anything before—not even student government. The learning curve was steep, and it was not easy. From fundraising to building a campaign brand, I had to go outside of my comfort zone and dedicate all of my free time to the campaign. Even though I still worked full-time as an SLP, I typically finished my work and Individualized Education Program (IEP) meetings by 4:00 p.m. and had sufficient time to spend my evenings doing campaign work.

Not long into the campaign, a primary challenger entered the race. He had experience as an elected school board member, city council member, and state legislator. Many referred to him as a "political animal." I kept focused and continued sharing stories about students and educators as a way to highlight my priorities. "Mason" was featured often. I wanted the public to know the importance of special education and how speech therapy and so many of the critical services offered in our public schools changed the lives of children. Although many said that I lacked the political experience to win an election, I felt strongly that the leader of the state education agency needed to be an educator with direct classroom experience, rather than a politician.

The competition began to heat up between me and my primary opponent, and we were invited to be the featured speakers for a "forum" during a luncheon. The event organizers said we would each be asked the same questions so that the audience could learn the ways in which our views differed. I had to take time off from work to make the event, but it seemed like a worthwhile opportunity to share my story as they expected a large audience.

When I arrived, the organizers explained more of the expectations. Not only would we each be asked the same questions, but there would also be an opportunity for rebuttals. I started to get a sinking feeling in my stomach as I realized what this event really was—a debate.

I am not a debater by nature. I had been dreading the day when I knew it would be unavoidable but this had caught me off guard, and I had not prepped or studied any debate strategies. I tried to keep calm and not reveal how anxious I really was. In front of approximately 150 people, I took my place with my opponent nearby, each with our own podium.

The questions were tough, and seemed to be intended to test our knowledge of nuanced education policy issues. The moderator asked, "What is your position on selling public land trusts to fund public education?" and I had no idea. Mortified, I did not know enough about the pros and cons to take a stance. My best option was to simply say that I wanted to do more research before taking a position and I yielded my remaining time.

The last questions were a blur. When it was finally time to pack up, I could feel my eyes watering and emotions surging up my chest. It was obvious to me that the audience members were gravitating towards my opponent's campaign materials and leaving mine behind. I felt like a failure and questioned my ability to continue as a candidate. Knowing I couldn't possibly drive home, I hid in a bathroom stall and tried to keep my tears at bay until I felt steady enough to leave. The doubts and every critique I had ever heard repeated through my mind, "Why are you even doing this? You know you're going to lose."

I had never so strongly considered quitting. It would be so easy to walk away, regain my personal life, and focus on my career as an SLP. I called my campaign manager Noah, a fellow teacher, and told him what happened. He listened empathetically and we talked through my options. We discussed the issues that I cared most deeply about and he reminded me that my educator experiences mattered in the race. I decided then that I wanted to continue on, to do deeper research so I wasn't caught off guard again, and to keep working hard through Election Day. At the very least, I knew I had more stories to share, stories about Mason, my colleagues, students and educators all across the state.

So I kept at it. I did my homework. I became a strong debater and beat the odds to win the primary election in August and then went on to win the general election in November of 2018. I was inaugurated as Arizona's superintendent of public instruction on January 7, 2019.

Just like my campaign, my inauguration speech was centered around my students. I was sworn in using my students' favorite book, *Too Many Moose,* and shared how speech therapy made a difference in Mason's life and many children like him.

It felt surreal to start my new career leading the Arizona Department of Education, and I was enthusiastic to get started.

In my first years in office, I have gained confidence as a leader. I am proud to be the first educator serving in this role in over 20 years and the youngest woman in the country elected to statewide office. While I advocate for children, I feel it is also important to be a role model for young women, especially aspiring educators and leaders.

I have had unique experiences to collaborate with and learn from many inspirational leaders, including the Phoenix City Mayor Kate Gallego, Navajo Nation President Jonathan Nez, and Secretary of Education Miguel Cardona. My work has afforded me the opportunity to travel out of state to attend conferences, present on our agency's achievements, and seek guidance from national experts on education policy.

I am passionate about my work because I see the difference that I make from the state level. Although there have been unexpected turns and new priorities due to the pandemic, I have continued to find ways to advocate for students with disabilities. From delivering an inaugural "State of Special Education" speech to the Arizona Legislature to allocating $500,000 to conduct a special education cost study, we are making gains in increasing funding and resources directly to classrooms.

Recommendations

1. Be brave to break out of the status quo to achieve your goals.
2. Identify at least a couple of mentors who have strengths in different areas to help answer your questions along the way, and ask for help when you need it.
3. Give the people around you a reason to feel hopeful and empowered to make a difference.
4. Develop a strategic plan with short-term and long-term goals.
5. Intentionally make time for vacations, exercise, and unplugging from technology for self-care.

My Wish for You

It's not easy to embark on a new leadership opportunity. I hope that you can surround yourself with people who provide encouragement and helpful suggestions.

There may be times when it feels lonely to take a new path, especially when some people may discourage you, but it's up to you to decide whether it's worth pursuing. As an SLP, remember to draw on your strengths in connecting with people, listening to community needs, and coordinating plans. Collaboration and building relationships are worth the investment of time to gain trust and make progress toward your goals.

My Community

Watch my interview with Mai Ling Chan: https://bit.ly/kathy_hoffman

Mouse over the QR code with your phone's photo app open to go directly to the podcast.

Ways to Connect with Me

www.electkathyhoffman.com

Twitter: @kathyhoffman_az

Facebook:
@electkathyhoffman

Kathy Hoffman is Arizona's Superintendent of Public Instruction and has led the Arizona Department of Education since her election in 2018. After working in special education as a school-based speech-language pathologist, Kathy ran for office to advocate for students and educators at the state level.

Still Listening

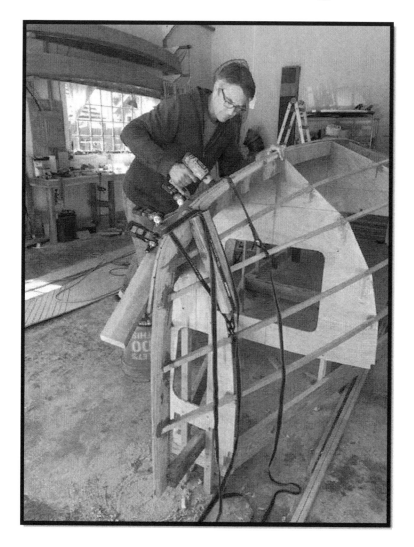

Chris Gibbons, PhD, CCC-SLP

Photographer: Eston Gibbons

* * *

"Tell me to what you pay attention and I will tell you who you are."

~ Jose Ortega y Gassett, philosopher and essayist

It is quiet in a desert canyon. Quiet because the canyon walls silence the unrelenting hum of life from the left and right. There is clarity in how discrete the parts are: river at the bottom, sky above, occasional bird flying, occasional other animal (rattlesnake, insect, deer, or rodent) making subtle noises along the canyon walls, scratchy but surprisingly fragrant scrub plants, and maybe a tree here or there. I learned to appreciate and seek that simple silence working as a river fishing guide before college.

Living out of a tent for three months each year, working long days cooking, cleaning, teaching customers how to fish, running dangerously rocky rapids, and making meaningfully trite conversation with people I hardly knew kept me busy. Every day was full and rhythmic with to-do's, and it took only a few nights sleep beneath the stars to forget what day of the week it was or what it felt like to ride in a car. About once a week or so I would dive into the cold water for a bath to knock off the dust and freshen up. Pretty good schedule for a young man trying to figure out who he was.

Whenever I had a few hours to spare, I would wander out of camp to find a trail leading up into the canyon. There I could find a good resting spot with a view and sit for long moments. From that vantage point I would stare at the rushing Deschutes River below, famous for steelhead and salmon fishing, white water rafting, site of the great railroad war of 1908, where ancient tribal marks of communication and art silently fade into obscurity upon mostly hidden rocks, and in which the lamprey eel remains abundant as it has for more than 450 million years—older than the dinosaurs. It is a rich and powerful heritage spanning the instant a fish rises to eat a fly, hatched only a few moments ago, to the unfathomably slow-motion effect of geologic epochs.

From where I sat, halfway up the canyon, the river was mute. No personal stories to tell. No ecstatic screams from rafters and rapids. No human history to reveal. No hint of life under the surface. Forever in miniature, it sat as a squiggly blue trail demarking the bottom of a V represented by its own undulating and shadowy desert terrain. Above where I sat, the canyon ridge looked like a cardboard cutout, stark and clear against a wide ribbon of summer sky replaced at night by a blindingly distinct star blanket. It was magic being halfway there, to and from, and finding a place in it all.

But that magic threw me off balance one day during my last year on the river when, enveloped by the scene before me, my mind wandered to what became a gnawing reflection that preoccupies me to this day.

It started with one of my siblings. As the two "younger kids" in the family, we were together a lot, and even from a young age I recognized that her life was radically different than most. She struggles with learning, emotional regulation, conceptual thinking, and motor planning. She looks at a river and looks at the sky and thinks about where she is–I mean, exactly where she is, looking down at the ground–not how the borders of her environment create a woven context or how the history of that place and the moment she is experiencing impacts her. For her, moments of reflection are rarely beautiful. She lives a different perspective and is encapsulated and tethered without having enough information to vault out of the physically immediate. It is difficult for her to see the bigger picture or build a vocabulary for thoughts and imagination that could sketch a more complete version of herself.

I realized then that her halfway point bore no resemblance to mine. Her halfway was encapsulated by a lack of knowledge and understanding. It was a place without yearning to know more about her surroundings because she literally didn't know how to describe the world beyond the immediate. She did not possess the vocabulary and conceptual tools to go there.

Staring at the canyon that day I suddenly wanted to stand up and call out to her and show her the place before me. I suddenly wanted to help her experience the joy of being part of a river and desert environment that marched forward unaware and unburdened by human psychology. I didn't have the clinical terminology then to describe where she was and what I wanted her to be. I simply yearned for my sister to gain perspective. To grow beyond the mental anguish of not knowing, of social isolation and teasing, phobias, and fear. To be halfway between what you know and where you are and feel curiosity and wonder instead of feeling stuck. How could I help her grasp the edge of a concentric circle further outside herself so she could be one step closer to experiencing a more fulfilling life? Was it too late now that she was a young adult? Did we miss our chance? I wanted a solution and I had no idea at the time that that moment of heartfelt yearning would so completely define my life trajectory.

I have always been a concrete guy when it comes to problem-solving. Broken chair leg? Get the epoxy and we'll fix it. Old car isn't running? Let's get the toolbox and start turning a wrench. Clothes dryer not working? I'll figure out what part we need. My attitude has always been that if someone put something together, I can certainly figure out how to take it apart and make it work again.

Nothing mechanical was safe at home when I was a kid. What started with toys became clocks, bicycles. Then I graduated to larger machines. During one summer I secretly disassembled, then reassembled, my parent's riding lawn mower, push mower, and rototiller while they were away at work. Frustratingly, I always ended up with important-looking extra parts after reassembly. But somehow, they all ran and mowed and tilled like the dickens for years. I am sure a few of those unidentified parts remain under my dad's workbench in the garage where I slid them with the side of my foot decades ago.

I learned quickly, however, that there was no manual describing how to fix my sister. Following that last year on the river, I went off to college to learn about the human condition and somehow make life better for people like her.

I had never heard of speech-language pathology until, after graduating, I found myself working in a group home for people transitioning from institutional care to residential placements. This was challenging for the people living there. They had quickly been relocated from the only reality they knew to somewhere entirely different with new staff and daily schedules. It wasn't going well.

After more than a few dramatic incidents and subsequent state oversight, a consultant was called in to help us gain control. It was all about control from our perspective. We wanted the residents of the house to be easy to manage, enjoy calm van rides, quietly watch sitcoms after meals, and always be cooperative during toileting. This was so far from reality that we willingly assembled on a Saturday morning, Dunkin' donut and coffee in hand, to learn from a specialist. We listened politely but were utterly unconvinced by her method. She claimed that the people in our care were not acting out with incompliant and sometimes destructive behavior because they needed restraint or medication. Rather, they were attempting to communicate with us. What we needed, she asserted, was a system for communication with which they could make their needs and emotions known so we could respond in-kind.

We stood together in the garage afterwards, hands in pockets and with raised eyebrows, incredulous.

"Head banging the wall until the drywall breaks is communication?"

"Throwing plates of food is communication?"

"Punching me and biting is communication?"

Things were out of control enough at that house that we grudgingly instituted the recommended program. We laminated photos and symbols and stuck Velcro on the walls to hold smiley and sad faces and had a rigorous daily checklist for data and comments. We began to only interact with each resident when we had picture-symbol support and choices available.

It changed everything.

A group home that was on the brink of closure with residents prepped for psychotropic medication transformed into a calm and collected household within weeks. We were stunned by the impact.

Here was something I could hang my hat on. This was a concrete solution. A way to open actual dialogue with people I had known for nearly a year, yet hardly knew in the ways that typically connect us socially. This was a method by which these residents could grow beyond cyclic and redundant frustration and, literally, live differently into the future. Like my sister, the people at that group home had been stuck halfway with no path forward and without a strategy to get them further. Unlike my sister, they had been provided with the first rung of a ladder. Hard to say how high they would climb, but it was definitely up and away from where they were.

Now I could envision, without detail, a life mission. Some people attack world hunger with every resource they can muster, for others it is preventable disease, clean water, or recycling. I began to march forward to replicate in as many ways as possible the success witnessed at that group home. With the right tools and approach, people could express and grow their personality, be freer to be known as an individual, and be less stuck. It was, and remains, a mission founded on human rights, dignity, equity, and social justice and I wanted to make as big an impact as possible in the time we have while darting across the surface of this planet. I never set out to lead. I was inspired to do something, to change things for the better with purpose and conviction.

I enrolled in the speech-language pathology post-baccalaureate program at Portland State University a few days after learning that our consultant was an SLP (speech-language pathologist) and augmentative and alternative communication (AAC) expert (incidentally, that SLP was Melanie Fried-Oken, who later became my clinical fellowship year supervisor, employer, friend, confidant, and lifelong mentor). She was recently inducted as an ASHA (American Speech–Language–Hearing Association) fellow and remains a powerful force of nature in AAC and her community.

I specialized as an AAC clinician early in my SLP career and have continued to dig deeper as a private practitioner, consultant, educator, researcher, developer, and manufacturer. I have experienced elation after implementing a life-changing language system with a child and wiped away tears of frustration and sadness when a client has made limited progress or a person with ALS (amyotrophic lateral sclerosis) has died before an AAC system was delivered that would have allowed critical communication with family at end of life. I have taught AAC courses to hundreds of graduate students and have been lucky enough to have been invited to assist on research with chimpanzees learning symbol communication, using a brain-computer interface with people who are functionally locked in, as well as other novel AAC techniques, language strategies, and clinical paradigms.

Several years ago I helped launch an iPad-based AAC device with AbleNet in an effort to help democratize the funded AAC marketplace while working with an esteemed group of colleagues, including Tobii Dynavox, PRC/Saltillo, Team Gleason, Medicare advocates, and others, to reestablish public funding for speech-generating devices.

Such varied experience has only left me hungrier to solve bigger issues in the world of AAC. I can see the problems laid out with maddening clarity, yet the solutions remain murkily in relief or inaccessible until we push technology and intervention to meet them. It is the classic Aristotelian problem of "the more you know, the more you know you don't know." That reality keeps me awake at night because I have now known for a long time that we can do so much better.

I am currently head of the U.S. division of Smartbox Assistive Technology, an AAC software and speech-generating device manufacturer. The U.S. AAC community is a remarkable group, and I am proud to be part of this moment of growth and awareness. We are no longer a cottage industry of engineers and tinkerers working in garages and basements using soldering irons and glue guns to build communication tools. We are infusing artificial intelligence, advanced language prediction algorithms, diverse symbol systems, and brain-computer interfaces into technology developed and built specifically for AAC. We collaborate with Microsoft, Apple, and Google. And yet, it still feels like we are chasing the bumper of the car while trying desperately to keep pace with consumer technology and expectations. It is a virtuous footrace, and I humbly accept the challenge.

In my position, I also accept the responsibility to shout about why it is so important to do what we do the right way; the people we are in service to and who define our purpose for what we do is at the top of our minds every day. I owe it to my sister.

She, along with millions of others like her in the United States and around the world, does not have the privilege or position in society to shout about such things. She does not identify or define her halfway points. She has always kept me from feeling stuck or following along without question or intention. Spurring me to shoot ahead for the next halfway point and begin pushing a new envelope, dragging as many people with me who are willing to listen.

With every leap as an SLP, I feel like I keep relearning the same thing, broadcast to me on some imaginary screen in my head while the colors become more vibrant with each iteration. It seems so simple on the surface: Our job is to conceptualize and scaffold opportunities for participation. Whether that is by way of phonology or morphology or deglutition or motor speech or paradoxical vocal fold dysfunction therapy or social skills or fluency or AAC or the 45 other things we address, our goal is to increase opportunities.

For me, in my specialty area, that job description reiterates daily how much further we must go before we can claim we've fixed anything. The person who can access a computer with their eyes but is unable to send an email as easily as the rest of us continues to be disenfranchised. The person using a switch to scan through activities to make choices for play who is not also being taught basic syntax or literacy skills is being told they have limits. The person using an iPad to express their feelings without their communication partners responding appropriately is left halfway between knowing and being.

As SLP professionals we have an opportunity to be relentless in our advocacy for all our clients. We should feel like a stick is constantly at our back pushing our comfort level because we know enough to know better than to be comfortable or complacent. Few other professions allow for such a natural mingling between how we live 24/7 and how we express ourselves professionally. With an authentic acceptance of that privilege comes joy, satisfaction, and positive inertia that can fuel your journey as far as you allow.

Recommendations

1. Define, then redefine, what constitutes equity for your clients.
2. Listen every day to the people we serve, their families, and our colleagues so our decisions are made in context.
3. Inform that context to help define each client's halfway point and progress milestones so it stimulates their healthiest perspective possible.
4. Be critical of our profession to be a voice for constant improvement. We are so very far from being done.

"The outcome of doing nothing is predictable"

- Anonymous

My Wish for You

When I was asked to contribute to this book, I immediately responded with an appreciative "yes" and then, almost as quickly, began to wonder what I might offer. I am certainly no more special than any one of you and far less special than many.

What I have learned that is valuable to me is something I have observed that we all do every day but often goes unrecognized. That is, by having chosen to do what we do, or in my case was inspired to do because of my sister, we express deeper motivations that drive us to care, to insist that everyone has a right to participate, to accept the responsibility that our role, without excuse, is to be the best resource possible to that end. So much of who we are is a result of what we experience, what we are taught, and what we have the capacity to process and take on as our own.

My wish for you is that you represent, as a person and as an SLP, a nexus point for solutions in ways few others can, and to thereby lead with heart, focus, and passion.

My Community

Watch my interview with Mai Ling Chan:

https://bit.ly/chris_gibbons

Mouse over the QR code with your phone's photo app open to go directly to the interview.

Ways to Connect with Me

chris.gibbons@thinksmartbox.com

www.linkedin.com/in/chris-gibbons-

https://thinksmartbox.com/

Chris Gibbons has worked in a variety of clinical, research, and industry settings as a private practitioner, educator, assistive technology specialist, and policy-level consultant. For the past few decades, he has focused solely on advocating for and contributing to AAC-user success through increased access efficiencies and by working to improve funding for speech-generating devices.

You Become What You Believe

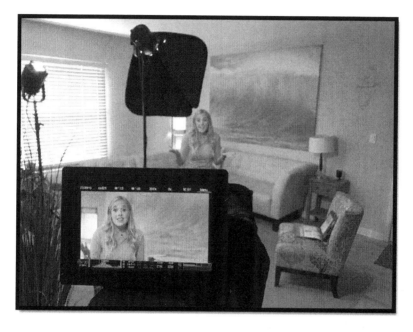

Rachel Madel MA, CCC-SLP

* * *

I sat alone in a Trader Joe's parking lot with mascara running down my cheeks and my head just as messy with worry. I was 29 and had just sold nearly all of my belongings on a whim and moved to Los Angeles.

Had I just made a huge mistake? Could I actually pull this off?

I never would've anticipated relocating to L.A. from my home state of Pennsylvania, but in 2014, it felt like the City of Dreams was calling me. I hopped on a one-way flight, determined to answer one question: How can I make a greater impact on a larger scale for children with severe disabilities?

The first step in my plan: Start a private practice.

I naively assumed that building a private practice would afford me the time and financial resources to work on my big-picture plan. Naive, because I had no concept of how much energy and effort it would actually take to build a successful speech therapy practice. I also had no clue what this "big-picture plan" of mine actually looked like.

As a fledgling entrepreneur, I really had no idea what I was doing. So I did what every grown woman does when faced with a problem: I called my dad. Every single day.

My first year living in Los Angeles was a straight hustle (Cue Rick Ross's song "Everyday I'm Hustlin"). I was attempting to balance all the necessary foundations of building a successful practice: solidifying relationships with potential referral sources; establishing a reputation for strong clinical skills, and optimizing the operating procedures within my business so I could spend time building my caseload instead of administrative tasks.

My stress was at an all-time high and I remember frequently being jolted awake at 3:00 a.m. in a cold sweat wondering if I'd have to fly back to the East Coast and live on my parent's couch. During those initial days, my dad served as a sounding board for business ideas and a crutch when I felt like I didn't have the courage or stamina to keep going. We spent hours on the phone, typically while I was sitting in a

Trader Joe's parking lot, killing time between clients. Together we brainstormed what kind of business model I could create that was scalable and could generate the greatest impact. I look back on that time and remember vividly how lost I felt. If only something or someone could give me clarity so I could devise a plan and start executing it.

An apparent theme emerged in these parking lot talks: my fear of failure. One rainy day, with a half-eaten bag of Trader Joe's peanut butter pretzels on the passenger seat, I lamented to my dad about my lack of clarity. I had dozens of ideas, but seemingly no idea where to focus my energy.

I'll never forget his words: "The only person standing in the way of your success is YOU." His words stung at first but began to resonate with me. It was at that moment I realized my indecision and inaction was stemming from an intense fear of making the wrong move; I was paralyzed by the fear of failing.

Even now, seven years later, I still circle back to my dad's words when I'm feeling stuck and question whether fear is the hidden culprit behind my internal struggle. His words also sparked my curiosity in the immense power of belief, both in myself as well as in the clients I serve.

"Believe they can, and they will."

This message adorns a slide I share at the end of almost every speaking engagement because it's the single most important takeaway for educators.

As a speech-language pathologist who specializes in augmentative and alternative communication (AAC), every day I'm working closely with individuals who have complex communication needs. Some have neurological conditions, some have genetic conditions, some have severe physical disabilities. For all within this population, communication is a significant challenge. By the time families come to my practice to explore AAC, their child has typically been in years of speech therapy with little to no progress. Too many times, I've sat across from teary-eyed parents, listening to their journey with doctors and educators who said their child will never communicate. Many parents lose hope that their child will ever learn to connect with the world around them.

I've learned that the act of believing in a child's potential is the most powerful gift you can give. Without adopting this fundamental belief, our children can't possibly reach their fullest potential.

In 2017, my passion for AAC took me 8,000 miles from Los Angeles to Phnom Penh, Cambodia, where I partnered with a nonprofit working to increase access to speech therapy. During my two-week trip, I spent time working alongside therapists teaching the fundamentals of AAC. My time in Cambodia was powerful, particularly an experience I had with a 17-year-old autistic student, Keo.[9]

Before heading to Cambodia, I collected a handful of used iPads to donate to the organization. I told the clinic's director to choose four students who they thought would benefit the most from a high-tech speech-generating device, and Keo was at the top of the list for an AAC assessment. The director believed he had enormous potential for communication if the

---

[9] The student's name was changed to protect his identity.

right technology was in front of him. The family was so eager for the assessment that they traveled four hours from their rural village to meet with me.

On the day of the assessment, Keo walked nervously into the therapy gym with his family, his head down and gaze locked on the floor. After showing him a few animated videos on YouTube, his demeanor eventually relaxed, and he started communicating. Keo had a small vocabulary of words in both English and Khmer (Cambodia's official language) to communicate. He demonstrated significant challenges formulating his thoughts into more complex sentences.

As we paged through a book he had chosen from the waiting room, I quickly realized Keo had very few verbs in his repertoire to describe what he saw. Verbs are the glue that hold sentences together, so it was no wonder he had trouble formulating his thoughts beyond single words.

I quickly drew three boxes on a piece of paper: WHO + DOING + WHAT. We practiced this formula for 15 minutes as I helped him learn to navigate his way through the device to build two and three-word sentences. Finally, I pulled up a picture scene of a duck pond to see what he could do on his own. He hesitated at first but then slowly began navigating the iPad, carefully tapping words to craft a message: "Duck jump at water."

As we sat across the table from one another, our eyes locked and huge smiles spread across our faces. He looked up at me proudly, and I'll never forget his face. It was a simple sentence, and yet the room buzzed with energy and amazement. In that moment we all realized the power of technology to unlock Keo's communication. It all began with presuming he had that potential inside of him in the first place.

Watching Keo so quickly learn to communicate through an iPad was an extraordinary moment, but my mind kept circling back to this nagging thought: If Keo could learn how to communicate so quickly, imagine if he had been introduced to AAC when he was in preschool. Where would he be now? How would his life be different if he had 15 years of consistent access to communication?

I spent the remainder of my time in Cambodia traveling solo and reflecting on the powerful experience I had volunteering. Clarity finally began to emerge as new questions compelled my unique gift to reveal itself. How could I help more students like Keo gain access to AAC? How could I inspire the belief in every child's potential to communicate? This experience abroad ignited my passion in making a greater impact and, ultimately, was how my online business was born.

"Welcome to Talking with Tech, my name is Rachel Madel..." I practiced it over and over again with a shaky voice and sweaty palms as self-doubt circled in my mind. What kind of false advertising had compelled Lucas Steuber (you can read his story in the second book in this series, *Becoming an Exceptional AAC Leader*) to ask me to co-host a podcast about AAC? I was not an AAC expert and barely knew what a podcast was.

Waiting in my Zoom meeting, I did some background research on my interviewee, Ajit Narayanan. He is an award-winning inventor from Silicon Valley who created the AAC app

Avaz and did a TED Talk with more than 1.4 million views. No pressure.

Luckily, I had received my undergraduate degree in journalism, prior to shifting gears and pursuing my master's degree in speech-language pathology (a career shift inspired by an encounter with a little boy with special needs who was being bullied, the choice to stand up for him, and a funny story of how I actually got into grad school... but those are stories for another day and another book).

Despite my 10-year hiatus from journalism, I was praying that my interviewing skills came back as easily as my bike riding skills. After I introduced myself to Ajit, I took a deep breath and hit the record button. I focused on my scribbled post-it note of questions while simultaneously playing the role of pro podcaster. Relief washed over me once the interview concluded, and I was thankful I survived my first ever podcast recording unscathed.

Over the course of the next year, I arrived at every podcast recording a little less intimidated and a little more sure of myself. I gave myself mini pep talks in my bathroom mirror and practiced my intro and outro on repeat. Our podcast reach was small at first, but quickly grew over time.

I'll never forget the first time I was recognized by a stranger. I was walking down the hallway at a conference and heard, "Oh my gosh, are you Rachel from Talking with Tech?!" After a quick selfie with my fangirl, my head was so big it could barely fit out the door. I continued to meet listeners of the podcast and read their emails, messages, and reviews and began to realize the impact our niche podcast was making.

Since we launched the podcast in 2017, the *Talking with Tech Podcast* now has almost half a million downloads with listeners in more than 100 different countries. We've interviewed leading researchers, clinicians, parents and AAC users themselves to discuss how to best support individuals who use AAC. Every week I get to have a mini professional development/therapy session with my co-host, Chris Bugaj. Together we share our clinical experiences, troubleshoot our biggest AAC challenges and celebrate our small wins along the way. The podcast has quickly become a well-respected platform, creating a powerful sphere of influence with a long ripple effect and giving multitudes of children access to technology that can open up communication and connection.

The evolution of the podcast hasn't come without internal struggle, and I've shared this to emphasize you don't always realize what's going on behind the scenes. If you listen back to the very first episode of *Talking with Tech*, you likely wouldn't realize I was secretly terrified, had a knot in my chest, and felt like a complete imposter the entire time. When being asked to start a podcast, it would've been easy for me to succumb to my inner critic planting seeds of doubt in my head. After all, I didn't have any experience in podcasting and could've easily rationalized my decision to turn down the opportunity. In those times of self-doubt, the words of my dad continued to ring in my ears: "The only person standing in the way of your success is YOU."

Any type of transformation, big or small, starts with the unwavering belief that change is possible. Throughout my journey as a speech-language pathologist, I've realized that one of my gifts is believing this for all children, even those with the most complex disabilities. I am the champion of this belief for the families I serve because this belief is contagious, and it's the seed that can help a child grow to reach their truest potential.

I've also recognized how holding onto the positive power of belief can deepen my relationships, both professionally and personally. I practice arriving to conversations with an expansive energy that encourages others to dream big and take risks. We need more people in this world brave enough to share their experience and turn ideas into action.

The most important skill I've developed is to question when my mind starts replaying a narrative of self-doubt and roadblocks me from achieving my goals. When I get trapped in this downward spiral, I gently remind myself I am capable of anything I set my mind to. Perhaps this belief starts with a repeated message from a parent or teacher or therapist, but over time we can learn to cultivate this belief until it becomes our own truth. And that's the most beautiful gift we can give ourselves and the world.

Recommendations

1. **Start before you feel you're ready**. You can make up a million reasons why it's not the right time to start a business or to take a risk and try something new. For so long, I used my "lack of clarity" to justify why I wasn't taking action, and I ended up wasting a lot of time. Start turning your ideas into actions and remember that you can refine and improve as you move forward. The key here is that you're moving. Don't let perfection stand in the way of your progress.

2. **Focus on who you're helping.** I made the mistake of desperately trying to create a business that would be

"successful" instead of focusing on who I was serving and how I was helping them. It's easy to get caught in the comparison game and try to replicate the success of others. Really start listening to the customers you're serving, and design your offering around the feedback you're getting from them. Once I started prioritizing who I was helping and made that my central focus, everything else started falling into better alignment.

3. **Outsource tasks that don't serve you.** Like every bootstrapping entrepreneur, I started my business as a one-woman show. I quickly learned that in order to scale and grow, I needed to hire a team to help with tasks I didn't like or have enough expertise in. Prioritize where your energy is best spent and quickly outsource simple tasks that are draining you. If you invest money on outsourcing, you afford yourself the time to focus on scaling your offering. The more your business grows, the more money you have to funnel back into your business to keep growing. Instead of focusing on working IN your business, focus on working ON your business.

My Wish for You

Believe there is something greater inside of you than any obstacle you might face. Fear is simply a sign that you are taking risks to learn and grow. Big success rarely comes without stepping out of your comfort zone. Lean into the discomfort, and remember that confidence is built slowly over time and through an accumulation of successful experiences. If you have an idea, lead with sharing it because you can't even imagine the impact it might have.

My Community

Watch my interview with Mai Ling Chan:

https://bit.ly/rachel_madel

Mouse over the QR code with your phone's photo app open to go directly to the Interview.

Ways to Connect with Me

www.rachelmadel.com

www.instagram.com/rachelmadelslp

www.facebook.com/rachelmadelslp

www.talkingwithtech.org

Rachel Madel is a Los Angeles-based speech-language pathologist and AAC expert dedicated to coaching parents and professionals on how to incorporate technology to best support speech and language development. Rachel presents both nationally and abroad on using technology for children in classrooms and at home to support communication skills. When she's not working with children in her private practice, she co-hosts a weekly podcast called "Talking with Tech" that focuses on best practices in using technology to support communication for children with complex communication needs.

Hope Speaks the World's Language

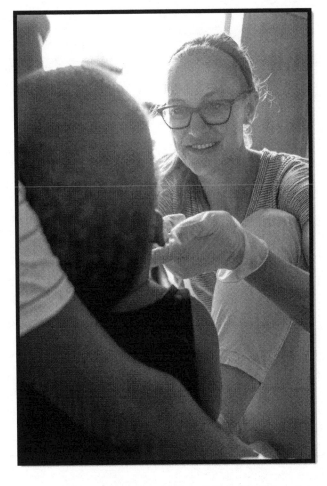

Kari David, MA, CCC-SLP

Photographer: Candice Lassey

* * *

On any given day, living in Uganda requires constant flexibility.

We plan out our weeks with therapy, mentorship, meetings, and community events, expecting that about 50% might go according to plan. We are forced to reassess, adapt, respond, repeat. For an American SLP (speech-language pathologist), who typically loves a good planner and organized schedule, the unpredictability rocked me for my first few months in Uganda. I felt like I had lost my balance, never knowing what was two steps ahead.

But over time, I learned to adjust and plan out my days, adding a lot of extra time for stops along the way and conversations with families. Here, it's never just a "hi" in passing but always an exchange of "How is your family," "Thank you for the work," and checking in on life. I've learned to honor these moments because these daily conversations frequently lead us to stories of people living with disabilities. A question from a community member about where we are heading can lead to a neighbor bringing us to the home of a child who has been hidden away out of fear that they may be harmed because they are differently-abled.

One such occasion was on January 15, 2016, when I went to Katanga slum to do our regular therapy in Mama H's home. Over the past few months, she had become a true champion for children with disabilities living in this community. Each week, Mama H would find children who were being hidden away and invite their mothers to come to our next speech and language therapy session at her home. On this particular day, we met a child named "C."

When we walked into Mama H's house, we found C curled up in the smallest space between the sofa and the wall of the dark 10x10 foot home. This was the first time she had seen daylight and been in contact with other people. She was rocking back and forth with her head crouched between her knees, gently tapping her finger and visibly fearful of this new situation. Mama H shared that C's mother had left their family when C was three years old because of the stigma associated with having a child with a disability in Uganda. To keep C safe from people who may want to harm her, or even kill her, because of her disability, C's dad locked her in their home each day while he went to work to provide for their family. For 10 years, C spent her days at home, isolated, without any social interaction.

At this moment, the social worker and I were overcome with feelings of helplessness. "Where do I even begin?" I thought to myself. How do you start to engage with a 13-year-old child who is completely overwhelmed by the sights and sounds of a whole new world that she is trying to process for the first time? I moved closer and stretched out my arms. She cautiously leaned in and sat close, and we slowly rocked back and forth. Mama H started to sing and we saw C's body begin to calm. In moments like these (moments which we encounter way too frequently), my heart rages.

How, in 2021, is this injustice still a reality for the millions of people living with disabilities around the globe? And how is it that most people are unaware about the hardships that people with disabilities in developing countries face? Being with C reminds me how much more work is yet to be done globally, both for the empowerment of the child and for the empowerment of parents to be brave and break from culturally sensitive norms marking people with disabilities as a curse.

One of the greatest challenges my husband Ben, who is also the country director at Hope Speaks, and I have faced over our six years in Uganda is the overwhelming amount of need. Community needs. Therapy needs. Financial needs. Organizational needs. Family needs. Personal needs. At the end of the day, the needs are always greater than what we can meet. My capacity as one person will never be enough. At times, I get stuck in this place of feeling overwhelmed and feeling inadequate. When we are faced with injustice and bear witness to the situations and stigma faced by people with disabilities, it can feel like no matter how much we do, it will never make a significant impact. Our attempt at making any sort of change seems like a drop in the ocean in comparison to how much work is still to be done. The vastness and severity of the need can, at times, overshadow the small glimpses of hope and the passion that we had when we first started.

But in these moments, our tribe steps up and our faith in something greater than us comes into play. Our Ugandan team, our passionate therapists, our board of directors, our friends, our family, our church partners, our donors. They show up like the Red Cross, ready to jump in and share the load. They pray, they give, they treat, they advise, they encourage, they donate, they advocate, they volunteer. Our tribe shows up in a thousand different ways to remind us that although we may feel isolated (especially in the middle of a pandemic!), we're not forging this path alone. Each day, they remind us and each family we serve that there is a global community of people who care—and that they'll do everything possible to make sure that every child has a voice and that each voice is heard.

The truth is, even if for all our work only one precious child had a better life, it would be worth it. But when we take a step back, we see thousands of children, families, and community members who have felt the effects of our tribe. From the Kantanga slum to Kasokoso, across Uganda, and around the world. Speaking out in big ways, and small ways, embracing the idea that each child has been created perfectly for a brilliant purpose that the world deserves to witness. In times of great need when we encounter indescribable suffering and injustice, we focus on the light. The small glimmer of hope in a smile or a "mama" uttered for the first time. Each spark is a sign that hope is around each corner, if only we just pause to make space for it. This hope speaks loudly, inspiring one family and the next and the next . . . until every child has a voice and until every child is celebrated for exactly who they were created to be.

Throughout my undergraduate and graduate studies, I questioned if speech-language pathology was what I was supposed to do with my life. So often I felt like I didn't fit the SLP mold, and I wondered if I should pursue a different major. I always felt this pull to work with low-resource communities, and when I started dating my husband Ben in college, I wondered how I would ever be able to use a degree in speech-language pathology if we were to move back to his home country of Uganda. I spent many hours in our university's career counseling office and enrolled in an introduction to education course to see if that would be a more "practical" fit for doing global work. I had always heard of doing medical or teaching work abroad but had never heard of opportunities for doing speech therapy internationally.

When I talked about my fears with Ben, I said, "If we ever move to Uganda, I'm going to be completely useless as a speech pathologist." He responded with, "I'm sure God will use your gifts somehow." At that time, he also had no clue how I could use speech pathology in Uganda, but secretly he was praying that by saying that, I wouldn't break up with him over my mini-life-crisis! I continued following the still, small voice inside of me, the one pushing me to follow through with this degree.

Two years later in 2014, as I was beginning my clinical fellowship at a small therapy center in Grand Rapids, Mich., Ben received a call from a close friend in Uganda who was the director of the orphanage in which he grew up. He told Ben they were in need of speech and language therapy for two children with special needs living at the orphanage. They had been looking for an SLP in Uganda for two years and only found one therapist whose waiting list was a mile long. At that time, the SLP was only seeing children one time every 18 months for therapy. He asked us to pray about moving back to Uganda to help these two children, but Ben quickly responded with a "No thanks, but I can do some research, and I'm sure I can find you an SLP there." We started researching, and what we found was devastating.

At that time, more than 3 million children were living with disabilities in Uganda. There was a huge shortage of speech pathologists in the country, with only two currently practicing in the entire nation of 40 million people. People with disabilities in Uganda face incredible hardship and stigma because they are differently abled. They are thought to be cursed, and as a result, they are at high risk for being abused, locked away, and even killed. We talked with people on the ground and connected with other organizations working in the disability sector, and each conversation confirmed that the need for therapy services was great.

Our hearts broke when we heard about the situation, but it all seemed too daunting to address. We felt completely unqualified to make any impact whatsoever given the size of the need. We continued to live our normal life in Michigan. I was working at what I thought was my dream job, yet, over time, I couldn't get those two children off my heart and my mind. I was sitting in my therapy room one day planning a session, and I thought to myself, "if I leave this job, my clients will be moved to someone else's caseload, and they'll continue to receive the services they need. But Scovia and Caleb in Uganda would continue to wait for therapy—for who knows how long." At that point, after tons of prayer, we decided to move to Uganda.

In November 2015, we packed our bags and moved to Wakiso, a district in the central region of Uganda. I started by seeing around 20 children for therapy, and as time went on, our phones started ringing off the hook with additional families and organizations in need of therapy services.

In 2017, we started Hope Speaks, a registered nonprofit organization in the U.S. and Uganda, to expand our services, reach more families, and provide mentorship for Ugandan SLPs. Hope Speaks partners with children, their families, and communities to help them flourish and impact the world through speech therapy, advocacy, education, and social services. We use a holistic approach to address the needs of the entire family and community to target the stigma associated with disabilities, and set up support systems to help people of all abilities to thrive.

Today we have worked with more than 800 families around Uganda. Our goal is to make therapy services accessible to everyone in Uganda, regardless of their income level, by empowering Ugandans with the tools and education they need to be a catalyst for change in their communities and at a national level.

My favorite part of the work I do is those moments in therapy when I get to see parents connect with their children and catch a glimpse of their child's potential and how bright they are! It's such a blessing to have the opportunity to be part of their story, and not just doing the work of practicing sounds or forming sentences, but equipping parents with tools they can use to help unlock their child's potential.

Moving to Uganda and starting Hope Speaks has grown me in ways that I never imagined possible. Professionally, working in this context has forced me to think outside the box and take my creativity in therapy to the next level. When I first started out, I fit all of my pediatric therapy materials in a single bag. Each session was focused on using items that families could easily access or things they already had at home.

Doing therapy here has also stretched me in my clinical knowledge. From 2015 to 2017, our attempts to connect with other Ugandan SLPs were unsuccessful. There were no other SLPs in the country who I could brainstorm with or bounce ideas off of. On any given day, I would see a huge range of patients of all ages with a variety of disorders and communication challenges. Over 80% of my caseload consisted of children and young adults with severe cerebral palsy, a condition that I had never worked with during my internships or my first years working in the United States. Although I had the "book knowledge" from school, many of my nights were spent researching the best clinical interventions to address the new challenges I was seeing each day.

Starting Hope Speaks has been the catalyst for significant personal growth as well. For most of my life, I was extremely shy and introverted. Being in new situations gave me anxiety and my worst nightmare was any type of public speaking.

In 2015, something changed for me, and I found a new confidence in myself and in my calling. God gave me boldness for sharing our story and advocating for people whose voices need to be heard. I now stand in front of groups of hundreds of people and share about this passion that stirred within me to make sure that every child has a voice. Stepping out in faith and following the call to move to Uganda has unveiled a new strength I didn't know I had within me. It has grown my faith in God and shown me that there is a purpose for everything we experience in life, not only for myself but also for each of the clients and families we serve. When we hold our gifts, talents, and passions openly and selflessly, the world can be changed for the better. We never know what our small offering, our quiet "yes," will lead to. It's not about us or about me and what I can do on my own, but rather about the impact we can make when we come together and work to empower and lift each other up.

"I alone cannot change the world, but I can cast a stone across the waters to create many ripples." - Mother Teresa[10]

Recommendations

1. **Be confident in your calling.** Remember that you are created for this moment, and do something that only you can do.
2. **Find your tribe.** Surround yourself with passionate people who dream big and support and encourage you to do the same.
3. **Travel.** Get out of your comfort zone and see the world humbly with an openness to learn.

My Wish for You

My wish for you, at whichever point you are at in your SLP journey, is that you find your vocation–"the place where your greatest joy meets the world's greatest need," as American writer and theologian Frederick Buechner once said. The place where your passion wakes you up in the morning and keeps you going day after day, even in the moments when it all feels like too much to handle.

It's my prayer that your fear, like mine, will be replaced with boldness and confidence. The work you do doesn't need to be big to be important. Start with one small step to make the world a better place and then keep going.

My Community

[10] https://www.goodreads.com/quotes/4950 world-but-i-can-cast

Listen to my interview on the Xceptional Leaders Podcast with Mai Ling Chan:

https://bit.ly/kari_david

Mouse over the QR code with your phone's photo app open to go directly to the podcast.

Ways to Connect with Me

Website: www.joinhopespeaks.org

Instagram: @joinhopespeaks

Facebook: @joinhopespeaks

LinkedIn: @kdavidslp

Email: kari@joinhopespeaks.org

Kari David is the co-founder and director of Hope Speaks, an organization that provides speech and language therapy services and mentorship for SLPs in Uganda, East Africa. Hope Speaks works to increase access and availability of rehabilitative services in low-resource communities. Kari lives in Wakiso, Kampala, with her husband Ben and three children, Bridget, Shaluwa, and Judah.

Failing Forward

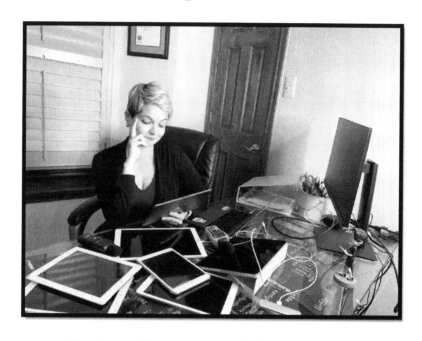

Barbara Fernandes, MS, CCC-SLP

Photographer: Jonathan Fernandes

* * *

Failure. It may not only be an unconventional first word in a motivational story, but also the most cliché one.

Failure is exactly what I am experiencing at this moment, a few months after releasing the biggest product for speech-language pathologists of my professional career because sales are far below expected numbers.

However, as I let the words flow, still feeling like a failure, I am taken aback by the strong sense that I was choosing to perceive sales numbers as the determinant factor for my success rate. Why? It makes no logical sense. Especially considering that I am not a sales professional: I am a speech-language pathologist.

As I sit here, reminding myself why I do what I do, I also understand what I have overcome to be sitting here, in my home office in Texas on a Sunday afternoon, writing a chapter in a book that will showcase the stories of many people I admire deeply. And, I am one of those people. Heck! I admire myself.

So, let's unravel how seemingly highly successful people on a journey full of ups and downs and failures, just like everyone, can still have enormous impacts on our profession.

I am now 38 years old and have not provided any type of speech and language evaluation or therapy to another human being in 10 years. By the age of just 28, I had already been running my own technology company for two years, one that created the very first app for speech therapists. Never in a million years could I have dreamed up the type of life I was living at just 28. That same year, I released at least seven apps on the App Store; I paid off all my student loans; I bought a boat; I nearly paid off my house, and my husband was able to quit his full-time job as a teacher to work with me on my business.

Around the same time, I was also being invited as a guest speaker to many state and international associations, universities, schools, and all sorts of private presentations, opening sessions, award ceremonies, you name it. I was doing what I absolutely loved and living the high life!

All of that sounds like quite the opposite of failure, right? You bet!

Would this become even more impressive if I shared that seven years before, I was counting my coins in Brazil to afford splitting lunch with my best friend? How does one go from being a monolingual Portuguese speaker in a developing country and walking to college because she doesn't have enough money to pay public transportation to having a professional bio that says trilingual speech-language pathologist ed-tech boss?

This is not an immigrant poster child story to show that anyone can achieve anything if they put their mind to it. This is a story of a risk-taker who, despite being afraid, jumped through every door that was opened to her by others before her.

My story is a story that could not have existed without a lot of other humans who opened or held my doors open and a system that allowed the daughter of a truck driver without any formal education in Brazil to become the first one in her family to attend a fully federally-funded college completely for free and where I could major in both speech-language pathology and audiology. While attending college, my father battled cancer, which caused our family finances to go from bad to worse. Making it to college every day and attending classes all day were my own battles.

In the midst of all this, a flyer caught my attention. I found out that, in partnership with the U.S. Department of Education, the Brazilian Department of Education was selecting students for an all-paid semester exchange student program in Pennsylvania. The program aimed to support Brazilian students in learning and eventually importing and implementing assistive technology back home. After a long and competitive selection process, I was one of four students to arrive at Temple University at the age of 21, full of dreams, hopes, and fears.

I will never forget being overwhelmed with powerful emotions the first time I walked into Temple University's library. I had never seen so many books in one place. I cried. That semester I learned about a new culture, a new language, all about assistive technology, and more. Speech therapy is the medium through which I learned English.

As the next door in my life opened, allowing me to transfer my credits to Temple and complete my undergraduate degree, I jumped through. As my English proficiency improved, so did my awareness of having a major shift in perspective from being a well-spoken communicator at a highly competitive university in Brazil to becoming a Latina woman with an accent seeking a degree in speech-language pathology. That experience definitely felt like a major downgrade.

That shift in perception could have made the mountain to the next step in my life impossible to climb. I experienced skepticism from professors, I was told that my accent was a communication disorder by the chair of the department, and the feeling of failure at such a young age was palpable. Yes! I thought about giving up and switching to a technology major many times. But that's not how my story was supposed to be.

Many women before me paved my way to allow me to graduate with honors, apply for my master's program in communication disorders with an emphasis in bilingualism, and be accepted with a full scholarship at Texas Christian

University. Let me take a few brag lines to say that in order to be accepted at that program, I needed to demonstrate proficiency in two languages I didn't speak two years prior: English and Spanish.

I am bragging now, but, back then, I was afraid. I felt like I didn't belong. I didn't belong in a class in which I was the only immigrant. I was the only one who spent the day speaking in either my second or third language. During that process, I experienced the biggest tragedy of my life to this day: the loss of my father. Once again, I didn't think I could go on. I was afraid, I was sad, and more than ever, I was lonely.

Becoming a speech-language pathologist, I realized, involved also discovering how to become myself in a whole new world, away from everything that felt "safe." To work through that realization, I took time off, I packed my bags, and set out to explore "speech therapy around the world." I left everything behind and postponed completing my master's program to find myself again. I spent three months couch-surfing through 15 countries and more than 40 cities throughout Europe. While sleeping at train stations, airports, or on porches, I got to meet, interview, and experience how speech therapists in Europe provided services to multilingual speakers. It was, on many levels, one of the most empowering experiences in my growing and healing process.

Three months later, I came back, graduated, and officially became a trilingual speech-language pathologist (SLP), which I proudly showcased on my graduation cap.

One year later in 2009, I officially filed Smarty Ears, my first business, with the State of Texas and launched my very first app on the App Store. At that point, in five years, I had moved to a new country, learned two languages, graduated with two degrees, and started a tech business. You would think I should be able to close my book and write THE END right then. Honestly, that was the part of the book that should be read "Once upon a time..." because my journey of becoming the SLP that fills my heart with joy was just beginning.

The first app I released was before the iPad was invented; convincing clinicians to allow students to touch their expensive iPhone 3 for therapy was in and of itself something that felt impossible to overcome. As time went on, app sales picked up, and I had recouped the money I had spent paying a programmer I hired off of Craigslist. In what felt like no time at all, the iPad was released, and app sales exploded. I started to believe that I had more than a business that would pay for my vacations as a school-based speech therapist. Once again, another door opened, and I walked right through it, leaving behind my full-time job as the bilingual evaluator at a school district to become my own boss. I was both proud and afraid.

Publishing anything—a book, an app, a resource, a blog, a social media post, or an Instagram reel—opens a part of yourself to the microscope of those who are ready to inspect your work under their lens. Publishing anything for speech-language pathologists is a dangerous place to put your self-esteem to the test. While I could tell you stories about how I felt when hundreds of colleagues at a national convention for speech pathologists and audiologists stood up and clapped after I demonstrated my latest invention—an app for articulation evaluation, the first of its kind, completely brilliant—I am here also writing about how I still, to this day, feel the weight of every criticism over my accent on demos, the rare overlooked typo, or the subjective choice of words on those apps. I know every SLP who wrote to Smarty Ears with their complaint didn't get to read about my struggles, my fears, or the other pieces behind the resource I made available to them. During Smarty Ears' first 10 years in business, I published more than 60 apps; each one of those apps is a part of me, a part of my gift to the world.

In those years, there were many ups and downs, wins and losses. Between the various "versions" of my apps released by other companies, blatant copycats, and the stress of learning to run a business, I kept looking for and finding open doors. Most of the open doors I had to go through were not like the massive, life-changing doors I exposed in previous paragraphs. Many of these new doors involved sleepless nights pushing through an emergency app update while also caring for a newborn baby; learning how to run and operate a business with nearly no employees; hiring and firing people; encountering endless mom guilt moments; supervising a clinical trial project way beyond my level of comfort and expertise; deciding which business partnerships were not a trap, or simply keeping up with the never-ending customer requests and support. Not to mention the learning curve of properly addressing men, who, in a primarily female industry, were still, in large, the ones founding and running SLP businesses and approaching my husband to discuss business dealings, although it was always clear who the boss was.

Just as I thought my learning curve had reached its peak, I was pushed to walk through another door and forced to establish two separate business entities.

Five years after filing for the formation of Smarty Ears in 2014, I formed my second business, Smarty Symbols. Smarty Symbols is a child of Smarty Ears; it was the graphic design heart of my previous four years of work, a child that needed to walk on its own.

Smarty Symbols is yet another way in which you will find my soul, my passion, and what brings me joy. It is another way in which I can bring my values into my profession.

I remember the moment I questioned why all the symbol representation for communication appeared to be this "colorless," male stick figure. It weighed heavily on me that I didn't want my symbol representation set to be yet another "colorless," male stick figure, so I came up with the "symbol of choice" idea to bring diverse representation to communication and visual support, something non-existent in any previous symbol set on the market.

As the owner of still small businesses, I take pride in knowing that the industry followed suit in the years that followed. Yet I can't help but also feel a little bit of something—that I will never be recognized as the person who made this impact, because just like in any industry, bigger businesses will always take the ideas and innovations of small businesses and make them their own. Ultimately, it is the pride of knowing that I raised the standards in this aspect that matters: Knowing that little people like you and me with big ideas can change the world one symbol at a time; seeing hundreds of photos of the Smarty Symbols in homes and classrooms around the world, and knowing that, in many places around the world, children with communication disorders communicate by clicking on a picture symbol set I envisioned and designed with my team.

Despite the fact that I have always made sure that most of Smarty Ears apps were available in Portuguese and Spanish, in addition to English, without any financial benefit, Smarty Symbols is where I walk right back to the door that brought me to the U.S. I keep pushing for diversity and having a symbol set now available in Portuguese and seven other languages.

Smarty Symbols and Smarty Ears are proof that investing in people works! My story does not have to be a one-off story if we give people the opportunity to perfect and express their gifts.

People often ask me if I miss providing direct services to children with communication disorders, which is the reason I studied for eight years (four in Brazil and four in the United States). My answer is that becoming an SLP brings me joy every single day, but I understand that my talents led to a different purpose in my profession—one that didn't quite exist before me. Despite having followed many roads, walking through opened doors, I ultimately paved my own unique path in my profession. It brings me joy to use my talents to create resources that will be used by my colleagues, who use their own unique talents to assist children and adults with communication disorders. My work already has and will touch the lives of many that I will never meet, hopefully long after I am gone. In following what brings me happiness, I am able to do what I love and what I am good at, while creating something the world needs and paying my bills with it.

Inspirational stories may be all about the hero, who despite all odds, succeeds in unimaginable ways. But my inspirational story is not just my story; it is the story of several people who have opened doors for me and the many others who created legislation for a federally funded college in Brazil, established an international exchange student program, presented at American Speech-Language-Hearing Association (ASHA) about the struggles of international students in communication disorders programs, invented the iPhone, and provided me with words and actions of support and encouragement through my journey. Those people are the reason a risk-taker like me can today be one more exceptional SLP.

May you also take risks to allow yourself to go through new doors, to be generous to open doors for others and kind enough to keep them open, to pave new ways in which speech-language pathologists can find joy doing their daily routine, or to fail just so you can succeed. As Oprah Winfrey says, "Keep failing forward."

Recommendations

1. **Be willing to get outside of your comfort zone.** This is where real growth happens, and most opportunities present themselves.
2. **Play to your strengths**. They probably represent your passions on some level, and your passion will be your driving force for moving forward.
3. **Don't kick down the ladder you climbed up on**. We all need help moving up. Don't lose sight of the people, the programs, or the legislation that helped your mobility and the needs of others to have similar opportunities.

My Wish for You

As you begin your journey, don't be overwhelmed by the thought that you need to have everything figured out. I had absolutely nothing figured out when I took my first steps, and the things I thought I had planned for all turned out either very different or much better. Focus on taking the first step, and keep walking.

My Community

Listen to my interview on the Xceptional Leaders Podcast with Mai Ling Chan:

https://bit.ly/barbara_fernandes

Mouse over the QR code with your phone's photo app open to go directly to the podcast.

Ways to Connect with Me

www.geekslp.com

Instagram: @geekBarbara

Twitter: @geekslp

Email: bfernandes@smartyearsapps.com

LinkedIn: https://www.linkedin.com/in/bfernanddes/

Barbara Fernandes, founder and CEO of Smarty Ears, is well known for her innovative and breakthrough product development, which translates science into user friendly and powerful technology to support individuals with communication disorders. Barbara transformed an entire industry to adopt mobile technologies through the design and development of over 60 mobile applications and an entire communication symbol library. As the founder of Smarty Symbols, Barbara also created the most inclusive and comprehensive symbol library and developed a powerful new technology that is disrupting the special education field by providing a platform for custom visual support creation. Most recently, Barbara has been awarded a small business innovation research grant by the National Institute of Health, and she released a ground-breaking technology called the Speech and Language Academy.

How I Became the Voice for Possibility

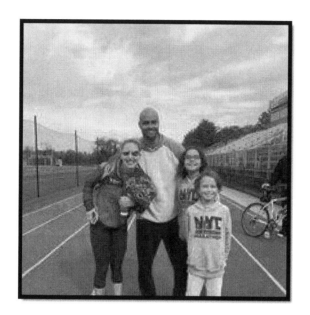

Nicole Kolenda, MS, CCC-SLP, PC

Photographer: Sally Ponce

* * *

I was set to launch my brand and podcast, the Voice for Possibility, on October 20, 2020. I had worked tirelessly during the pandemic on this while also homeschooling my children, teaching online for New York University, treating private clients via teletherapy, and running every day.

Although I had been running for years at this point, with three marathons under my belt, running during the pandemic took on a whole new meaning for me. I began training for the 2020 New York City Virtual Marathon in early July, and my run-streak was in full swing. Every morning I worked through my daily stress and pressures with each cumulative step.

The morning of October 20th was no different—except the "stress" I was processing on that run was from the biopsy I had of a lump found a few days earlier on my right breast. The day before, I rescheduled my podcast launch date (because the enormity of it all was a little too much for me to process) and set up a late afternoon meeting with my team to regroup. Three hours before that team meeting and five hours after my morning run, I got the call no one wants to get. I had breast cancer.

I was 44 years old and in the best shape of my life. I had recently gone vegan and I was running 60 miles per week. That moment is forever etched in my memory. My husband tried to console me, but I wanted no part of that. I didn't want him (or anyone else for that matter) feeling bad for me. I was in a state of shock.

Through tears, I explained to the women who had helped me get my website and branding to the perfect place and supported me in so many ways: The results were positive, and I had cancer. Saying it out loud sounded strange. Who was this person talking? Me? CANCER?

My husband and I decided we would tell our two children (8 and 9 years old at the time) that evening. I had my virtual marathon coming up in five days and I reasoned that if we told them the truth—that I had cancer and that I was fortunate to catch it early (Stage 1)—and then I went out and ran 26.2

miles at a local track, they would not think the situation was that dire.

I went on to tell my team that we were going to continue with my launch and that I was going to come out with my story. I had worked so hard for so long on both my website and podcast as well as my training for the marathon that I was not going to give any of it away to cancer. It was a bold move for me to share something so personal on social media, but the outpouring of love and support was incredible.

On October 25, 2020, five days after I received my breast cancer diagnosis, I ran the NYC Virtual Marathon—105 laps around a track—and set a personal record with a time of 3 hours and 43 minutes. There was a moment when I was out there running, around mile 25, when my hubby grabbed my children and they ran a bit with me. At this point, I was exhausted, and my legs were like butter, but I knew I was going to finish faster than I ever thought possible. I told my children to look at me—I wanted them to remember me strong.

I have always been a multi-hyphenate person, never quite fitting into any one mold. I have also always been into sports. I played volleyball at NYU while getting my bachelor of science degree in communication sciences and disorders. It is crazy to think that now, 23 years after I graduated with that degree, I am back on-campus at NYU, this time as the lead SLP (speech-language pathologist) on a National Institute of Health-funded treatment efficacy study. I am also an adjunct professor. Every once in a while, I look around and think, "Is this real? Am I really here?"

My mom instilled a strong push to be self-supportive. When given the choice between a wedding or college, she chose the wedding and made sure I would NEVER do the same.

My work ethic took shape when I was young. As soon as I could, I entered the workforce. From babysitting, to jobs at McDonalds, Rite Aid, Carvel, Anthropologie, Macy's, and Avis Rent-a-Car, I have always worked. These early experiences put me on track to open a private SLP practice on the Upper East Side of Manhattan once I had my master's degree and a bit of experience.

I loved the autonomy of my own practice, but I missed the professional collaboration, so I began teaching and supervising. I have worked at many wonderful universities in New York, but NYU wins my heart.

A pivotal point in my career came when I had children of my own. As a new mom in 2010, I began to approach my practice differently—treating the "whole child" now meant looking at the main caregiver(s) as almost an extension of the child themselves. I took to truly supporting the support system and the results were amazing.

I knew I wanted to explore this new-found role I seemed to have stumbled upon (although, as with most things in life, it actually was right there all along!), and I enrolled in the Institute of Integrative Nutrition. As a certified health and wellness coach, I can now FULLY support all of the moms who cross my path and further empower this community, to which I have dedicated my entire professional career.

Shifting my focus to the caregiver(s) came with many realizations. I learned that when the caregiver feels supported and the therapist can share the "weight" of the child's diagnosis in a meaningful and constructive way a beautiful thing happens–there is what I would call a "mindset" shift, and new possibilities avail themselves. The caregiver is given space to focus on themselves, which in turn, helps them physically feel better, which then gives them the ability to really "see" their child—not in comparison to other children or developmental norms—but simply as their child, with unlimited potential. There will also be an increased ability to handle any stressful situation that may arise, which is important because stress in life is inevitable, especially as the mama or papa bear to a child with a speech sound disorder. From this perspective, the caregiver no longer sees it as a "doom and gloom" situation (even though nothing has changed drastically with the child's diagnosis), and they now have permission to pursue some of their own passions.

I know firsthand the necessity for moms to find their own outlets and experience possibilities for themselves, separate from that of their child. As a busy mom and professional myself, I have found solace in running. Adopting the identity of a runner has been one of the greatest joys of my life–I have completed the NYC Marathon for the past 4 years (to date), and I love showing other busy moms that it is possible to have ONE thing that is solely theirs. As of this writing, I am currently training for the 2021 NYC Marathon, and I recently became certified as a Road Runners Club of America (RRCA) run coach!

This outlet has enabled me to find new possibilities within myself every single day.

By connecting daily with myself through running, I'm able to more fully show up for those I work mostly closely with, including children diagnosed with childhood apraxia of speech.

These children want to speak, but struggle to do so. Sometimes they are so frustrated with being trapped in their own thoughts that they lash out, understandably. The moment they produce a word not previously in their repertoire, when their eyes light up and they realize our work together is helping, that moment is everything. It also brings the bigger picture into focus for me. It helps to ground me when I am struggling with things in my own life. Expression is a human right that we can sometimes take for granted. Working with this population has both humbled and inspired me. They have also helped me shift my perspective.

Over the years, I have cultivated an "in the moment" mindset. I have come to realize, across all domains of my life, that to be successful and make progress we must be willing to take a good look at our mental, physical and emotional surroundings and "start where we are."

With my clients, I may want them to have better motor control or a more organized articulatory system, but I know I must meet them where they are (after doing a thorough diagnostic evaluation) and give them the support they need to attain their goals. In therapy, I am constantly re-evaluating the system to see what gains have been made; then I adjust. The same goes for teaching—I must meet my students where they are. If I am teaching a challenging concept, I know I have to start from the bottom and methodically work my way up, and then frequently check in to make sure everyone is with me.

Lastly, the breast cancer diagnosis and living through surgery and treatment has landed me in what I am affectionately referring to as "The After." I am not who I was; I am learning to accept who I am and what I am capable of. This has been particularly humbling with marathon training because my body is not the same. Although I wanted to start training at the rigor I did last year, with my target paces the same, I realized quickly I am still healing and I need to **start where I am** and go from there. One foot in front of the other. As I write this, my run-streak is at 270 days in a row. Before my surgery, on December 2, 2020, I ended my previous run-streak at 328 days. My goal is to get to at least 329 days in a row of running and take back the streak that cancer cut short.

While cancer shifted and cut short some things, I realize, in hindsight, how it also helped me expand in unexpected ways. One year after my diagnosis, I am in disbelief and filled with gratitude for all that I achieved in 2020–2021.

Not only did the podcast and website launch go well, we also came up with a five-day Pandemic Possibility Pursuit, a challenge for all of us (myself included) to continue to seek out and pursue possibilities in the pandemic. During those five days I shared different areas of my life that I was grateful for: family, relationships, wellness, career, and mindset. This led to the development of a Possibilities Playbook, a series of journal prompts designed to help the reader add more possibility to their own lives.

Curiously, too, although the podcast series and live Instagram interviews I did with each podcast guest were initially meant to help others, I was surprised to discover how important the wisdom embedded in them was to my own personal healing journey. Re-listening, I found each interview enlightening and witnessed my own growth and healing from the podcast series that I had meticulously planned out before my diagnosis. Isn't life funny that way?

During this time frame, I also wrapped up the teaching of my six graduate classes and graded all of the finals and papers. I executed Christmas in our household—with an epic design scheme and baked more than 1,000 cookies—mailing out five boxes to beloved friends and family across the United States, a joyful project that kept the semblance of normalcy for my children, and myself. And, we welcomed Isabella, a Shar-Pei puppy, to our family. Holding Isabella nine days after my surgery was a delicious gift.

What all of this continually shows me is how I've spent the last 20 years finding possibility in the sometimes seemingly impossible.

Whether it is with children looking to create their literal voices, graduates and clinicians looking to create new possibilities for themselves and those they serve, or women—especially moms—who feel alone and without a voice in their lives, I find a way to hold space for them. As a pediatric speech language pathologist, professor, mentor, runner, mother, and breast cancer thriver, I strive to be the voice of what is possible in every facet of my life.

Recommendations

Through my life and work experiences, ongoing education and mentorship, I share these personal recommendations with you as you create and grow your personal offering:

1. **Lean in to what makes you feel energized, even when you are exhausted**. I began to see early on that teaching lit me up in a way that made me feel alive. I love watching a student learn under my tutelage.

2. **Get comfortable ASKing questions.** I find myself saying this a lot to my students. I do not know what they do not know if they do not ask for clarification. Please—ask questions! It's the best way for your professor and others to understand how he or she can support you.

3. **Always keep your side of the street clean**. A mentor told me this once and it stuck. It means to do the right thing, so at night, you can lay down with a clear conscience. I always tell the parents of the children I work with the absolute truth, even if I know it is not what they want to hear. I do not lie or sugar coat anything. In the same vein, I give my students honest answers in class and tell my clients what they can expect from our time together. In short, I always keep it real, and that is why people have learned that I am someone they can trust. I do not take this lightly.

4. **Choose One**. My "Choose One" is running, but it really can be anything! The Choose One movement is about finding a goal. One goal that is solely yours. One goal that you do not feel guilty about or apologize about. One goal you commit yourself to accomplishing. We are so good at setting goals for our clients; we must learn to do the same for ourselves.

5. **Prepare for your Mile 19 Moment**. Mile 19 in the marathon is when I lose it. At this point in the race, you are so tired and your body is so depleted ...

sometimes, if you have not fueled adequately, your body even fails. This is affectionately referred to as "hitting the wall." In 2019, as I landed on Mile 19 of the NYC Marathon, I seriously considered taking a shot of tequila (I do not drink!) from a fraternity boy cheering from the sidelines. I was so tired that I convinced myself that I should quit (I just had to get through The Bronx first). It was irrational, and I knew it, and I was able to pull myself out of it because hitting the wall is expected. No matter how hard you train, a marathon is always hard. To prepare for your Mile 19 Moment is to understand that something could go wrong or your plan could hit a snafu and knowing how you will continue when those challenges arise. I repeated my mantra "you can do this," and that helped me stay the course.

6. **Do not be afraid to shine.** Remember, those who recoil when you go bright are not ready to hear what you have to say anyway.

My Wish for You

My wish for you is that you learn to appreciate the journey. The destination you think you are striving for will morph and change over the years, but the journey is where life is lived and lessons are learned.

I encourage you to cultivate multiple areas of interest—this will give you more joy in your life, which will in turn help you to be a better therapist. We are not one-dimensional.

If you do not already have one, start your own movement practice. This can be walking, running, yoga, biking, tai chi, or any other activity that gets your body moving. Movement is the biggest gift you can give yourself.

Lastly, learn what boundaries you must construct to keep yourself well and healthy. This could mean going to sleep at 10 p.m. every night or limiting time on social media. It could also mean not answering work emails on the weekend or after 6 p.m. I made the mistake early on of letting everyone have access to me, and honestly, it becomes exhausting. Because we are by nature caregivers, we want to help. But we must protect our own resources so we can give of ourselves in the best way possible.

My Community

Watch my interview with Mai Ling Chan:

https://bit.ly/nicole_kolenda

Mouse over the QR code with your phone's photo app open to go directly to the interview.

Ways to Connect with Me

www.nicolekolenda.com

LinkedIn: @nicolekolenda

Facebook:@nicolekolendaslp

Instagram: @nicolekolendaslp

Voice for Possibility podcast

Nicole Kolenda, MS, CCC-SLP, PC, is a New York state-licensed/ASHA-certified pediatric speech and language pathologist with over twenty years' experience working with children and young adults diagnosed with developmental differences. Nicole is an expert in pediatric motor speech disorders and is currently the lead SLP on an NIH-funded treatment efficacy study at New York University—where she is also an adjunct professor. Nicole is the founder of the inspirational Voice for Possibility podcast, a proud breast cancer survivor, marathon runner, and mom to two beautiful children.

Final Thoughts

I mentioned in the Introduction that 14 stories are only a small representation of the international community of speech-language pathologists who have already created or are currently immersed in the creation and growth of their immensely valuable offerings. That's because, although the opportunity occasionally arises, for the most part, SLPs (speech-language pathologists) are not often invited to share their "origin story" or inspiration for their achievements.

It is my personal wish that through this book and other available media, such as podcast interviews, blog posts, and in-person presentations, SLPs are spotlighted for the bummock—the portion of the iceberg that is submerged underwater—rather than just the public view of their story that everyone sees. It is through the age-old pastime of storytelling that we learn the humanistic side of challenge and accomplishment. Not everything is as simple as it seems on the surface. But through transparency, vulnerability, and courage to share, we learn the depth of experience and rainbow of emotions that people endure along their journey.

Have you enjoyed journeying with us? We hope so. Each story has been carefully selected from the myriad of experiences that make up our lives with the special intent of connecting with you. We hope that as you read each chapter you found instances of similarity— whether it was crying in your car, managing personal health issues, feeling helpless with a client, being inspired by a family member, exploring all the wonders of teletherapy, or any of the other realities shared. The most important thing to acknowledge is we are all human and only have 24 hours in our day. What makes us unique are our personal talents and life experiences that enrich our foundations. And, this book, alongside the other two volumes in this series, strives to represent the human essence hidden within the busy life of an SLP.

While most SLPs have the same basic courses in anatomy, physiology, articulation, and language, the choice to focus and prepare for either a medical setting or an educational one begins to set some of us apart. Others of us found it difficult to narrow down to only one track, and we created ways to include a mix of courses in both areas into our academic plan. Building on research and the tutelage of our professors, we completed our master's program with intensive clinical support from university staff as well as professional SLPs out in the field. This is only the beginning of our understanding of our true place within the profession and as an integral part of our client's team. In providing one-on-one services, we brought all of our past history; lived personal, cultural, and experiential experiences; and rich human essence to each interaction. Additionally, we are shaped by everything we've encountered and endured prior to and during our lives, and, in turn, that influences how we learn, how we provide services, and how we engage with our clients. For many of us, we are able to see gaps in the system or opportunities to improve, and this is where we begin to shine our true brilliance.

As you have read in our chapters, the co-authors are working to fill many widely different "needs." This includes unique technical resources to support clinical services, bilingual research and education, international clinical services, nonprofit organization, global education through a variety of media, advocacy through public service, clinical and staffing support, and individual recognition and support for the profession, to name just a few. And many more aren't represented in this book, including creative content creation to support clinical activities, multicultural advocacy, early intervention support for parents, deep-diving into feeding and swallowing services, supporting voice techniques for the trans and gender-nonconforming community, research across the continuum of age and diagnosis, and so many more!

But the beauty of our field is that we are not limited by our area of focus or by how we choose to serve. There is always the opportunity for a harmonious merging of our skills and talents with our passion to make a difference in the lives of others, and we have seen how exciting these offerings can be! From award-winning documentaries to successfully exited start-ups to state superintendent responsibilities to relocating and providing services in countries where people with disabilities are locked away out of public view, the need is great, and we are filling the gaps with our unique gifts and authentic presence. The exceptional, compassionate leaders spotlighted here continually show all of us that we are only truly limited by our own imagination and courage.

At the end of each chapter, we invited you to explore ways to expand your reach, and shared personal recommendations and pearls of wisdom we've earned along the way. These most certainly are not comprehensive nor are they guaranteed to bring you similar success, but they are genuine and heartfelt. Each co-author has taken time to reflect deeply on what has helped them in their forward progress, and what may have held them back. These private thoughts are openly shared with the unified vision of supporting you in your forward progression in all your endeavors. We also provide ways to contact, follow, and connect with each of us. This is because we truly believe that supporting each other is essential.

Here are a few more recommendations:

1. **Go beyond the speech pathology degree.** Add your personal talents, passion, and vision to the world of communication!
2. **Keep learning and expanding.** You can also find additional inspiration and support from co-authors of the previous books in this series; *Becoming an Exceptional Leader* and *Becoming an Exceptional AAC Leader*. Both books also include people who are dedicated to supporting people with disabilities and who have been inspired by personal lived experiences as well as through parenting and professional influences.
3. **Tune in to the wisdom all around you.** Listen to international voices and stories of global disability leaders on my Xceptional Leaders Podcast.

Thank you for taking the time to get to know us. Our collective wishes for you are that you find and walk the road to making your career as fulfilling as possible and that you increase your positive ripple effect in the world. Let us know how we can help you shine your brilliance and become an exceptional SLP leader.

Made in the USA
Columbia, SC
30 October 2021